Building Happier Kids

Stress-busting Tools for Parents

Hansa Bhargava, MD, FAAP

American Academy of Pediatrics
DEDICATED TO THE HEALTH OF ALL CHILDREN®

American Academy of Pediatrics Publishing Staff
Mary Lou White, *Chief Product and Services Officer/SVP, Membership, Marketing, and Publishing*
Mark Grimes, *Vice President, Publishing*
Kathryn Sparks, *Senior Editor, Consumer Publishing*
Shannan Martin, *Production Manager, Consumer Publications*
Sara Hoerdeman, *Marketing Manager, Consumer Products*

Published by the American Academy of Pediatrics

345 Park Blvd
Itasca, IL 60143
Telephone: 630/626-6000
Facsimile: 847/434-8000
www.aap.org

The American Academy of Pediatrics is an organization of 67,000 primary care pediatricians, pediatric medical subspecialists, and pediatric surgical specialists dedicated to the health, safety, and well-being of all infants, children, adolescents, and young adults.

The information contained in this publication should not be used as a substitute for the medical care and advice of your pediatrician. There may be variations in treatment that your pediatrician may recommend based on individual facts and circumstances.

Statements and opinions expressed are those of the authors and not necessarily those of the American Academy of Pediatrics.

Any websites, brand names, products, or manufacturers are mentioned for informational and identification purposes only and do not imply an endorsement by the American Academy of Pediatrics (AAP). The AAP is not responsible for the content of external resources. Information was current at the time of publication.

The persons whose photographs are depicted in this publication are professional models. They have no relation to the issues discussed. Any characters they are portraying are fictional.

The publishers have made every effort to trace the copyright holders for borrowed materials. If they have inadvertently overlooked any, they will be pleased to make the necessary arrangements at the first opportunity.

This publication has been developed by the American Academy of Pediatrics. The contributors are expert authorities in the field of pediatrics. No commercial involvement of any kind has been solicited or accepted in development of the content of this publication. Disclosures: The author reports a financial relationship with Freespira.

Every effort is made to keep *Building Happier Kids: Stress-busting Tools for Parents* consistent with the most recent advice and information available from the American Academy of Pediatrics.

Special discounts are available for bulk purchases of this publication. Email Special Sales at nationalaccounts@aap.org for more information.

Printed in the United States of America

9-471/0122   1 2 3 4 5 6 7 8 9 10
CB0128
ISBN: 978-1-61002-573-7
eBook: 978-1-61002-576-8
EPUB: 978-1-61002-574-4
Kindle: 978-1-61002-575-1

Cover design by Daniel Rembert
Publication design by Rattray Design
Library of Congress Control Number: 2021904849

Additional Books From the American Academy of Pediatrics

Achieving a Healthy Weight for Your Child: An Action Plan for Families

ADHD: What Every Parent Needs to Know

Autism Spectrum Disorder: What Every Parent Needs to Know

Building Resilience in Children and Teens: Giving Kids Roots and Wings

Caring for Your Adopted Child: An Essential Guide for Parents

Caring for Your School-Age Child: Ages 5–12

Co-parenting Through Separation and Divorce: Putting Your Children First

Family Fit Plan: A 30-Day Wellness Transformation

High Five Discipline: Positive Parenting for Happy, Healthy,
Well-Behaved Kids

My Child Is Sick! Expert Advice for Managing Common Illnesses
and Injuries

Parenting Through Puberty: Mood Swings, Acne, and Growing Pains

The Picky Eater Project: 6 Weeks to Happier, Healthier Family Mealtimes

Protecting Your Child's Health: Expert Answers to Urgent
Environmental Questions

Quirky Kids: Understanding and Supporting Your Child With
Developmental Differences

Raising an Organized Child: 5 Steps to Boost Independence, Ease Frustration,
and Promote Confidence

Raising Kids to Thrive: Balancing Love With Expectations
and Protection With Trust

The Working Mom Blueprint: Winning at Parenting Without Losing Yourself

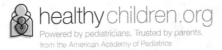

For additional parenting resources, visit the HealthyChildren bookstore at
https://shop.aap.org/for-parents.

What People Are Saying

Dr Bhargava's compassionate, informed guidance will help parents and kids reset their priorities, focus on health and happiness, and move away from jam-packed schedules, screen time, and stress. *Building Happier Kids* is an important resource for addressing the mental health crisis children are facing.

—Tanya Altmann, MD, FAAP, founder of
Calabasas Pediatrics and editor in chief of
Caring for Your Baby and Young Child

If you ask 100 new parents what one thing they wish for their children's futures, all 100 will answer, "Happiness." But then things get complicated—education, sports, social life, electronic media, financial pressures intervene—and the challenges of daily life overwhelm that simple wish. We and our children end up anxious, depressed, and exhausted—the opposite of happy. In *Building Happier Kids*, pediatrician, journalist, and mother Dr Hansa Bhargava maps the way back to our original destination, helping parents steer away from those ruts and dead ends and get back on the road to joy where we all started.

—David L. Hill, MD, FAAP, author of *Dad to Dad: Parenting Like a Pro* and coauthor of *Co-parenting Through Separation and Divorce: Putting Your Children First*

To my sisters, Dita and Aparna, who walk in lockstep with me and have forever stood by my side.

To my children, Ellora and Davik, who constantly give me joy, happiness, and gratitude for being a parent.

And to my mom, whose courage and love has taught me to be the best version of myself and that anything is possible.

Equity, Diversity, and Inclusion Statement

The American Academy of Pediatrics is committed to principles of equity, diversity, and inclusion in its publishing program. Editorial boards, author selections, and author transitions (publication succession plans) are designed to include diverse voices that reflect society as a whole. Editor and author teams are encouraged to actively seek out diverse authors and reviewers at all stages of the editorial process. Publishing staff are committed to promoting equity, diversity, and inclusion in all aspects of publication writing, review, and production.

Contents

Acknowledgments

As I look back at my journey in writing this book, I am filled with gratitude. I have been blessed by a caring community of people who helped me formulate ideas, guided me through the process, and provided incredible support that allowed me to turn my thoughts into a book for parents. I will not be able to do justice to all those who helped me but would like to try. I am greatly indebted to the families I have heard from and cared for over the years. These parents and caregivers have given me the privilege of caring for their children and shared their stories so that others could benefit. A special person in my life who truly impacted the writing of this book was my nephew Alec. Alec, a vibrant, young man full of love, battled mental illness for a long time, as well as substance use disorder. He tragically lost his life to fentanyl poisoning at the young age of 26. I've always known the importance of emotional well-being for our kids, but his untimely passing gave me the personal impetus to write this book for other families.

With utmost gratitude, I'd also like to thank the American Academy of Pediatrics (AAP) team, including Kathryn Sparks and Mark Grimes, for seeing the value in the idea of a mental health toolbox for kids and families. I am so appreciative of my editor, Kathryn, for her passion and commitment and for her tremendous advice throughout the process of writing this book. I am very grateful for the time that the various AAP reviewers, who are busy pediatricians themselves, spent reviewing my material for relevancy and accuracy, including members from the Council on Communications and Media, Committee on Adolescence, Committee on Psychosocial Aspects of Child and Family Health, Committee on Substance Use and Prevention, and Council on Environmental Health and Climate Change. I'd also like to extend my deep appreciation to the family engagement members who took the time to read the manuscript and provide invaluable feedback: Sondra Gilbert, Amy Holbert, Yovanni Millings, and Jodi Smith. I extend my utmost gratitude to Drs David Hill and Tanya Altmann, who were wonderful mentors to me. I could not be more thankful to Erin O'Donnell, a talented writer, who helped me put together several sections of this book. There were many colleagues whose advice was instrumental, including Colleen Paretty, former executive editor of *WebMD* magazine; Kim Richardson; and Liz Neporent.

Dr Linda Pak, clinical psychologist, and Dr Smitha Bhandari, child and adolescent psychiatrist, graciously gave their time to be interviewed about mental health illness and offered expert insights in this book. Dr Neha Pathak, a colleague, friend, and expert in climate change and lifestyle medicine, wrote excerpts in the fundamentals chapter, while Dr Michael Smith, my supervisor, gave me much needed encouragement and support. Dr John Whyte, author of *Take Control of Your Cancer Risk*, has been so generous in his advice and has shared his knowledge of writing books.

To spend time on a passion project in addition to your regular job, it is imperative to have leadership support you and encourage you to pursue your dreams. For this opportunity, I will forever be grateful to my boss, friend, and colleague, Kristy Hammam, former executive vice president of WebMD. Not only was she an incredible mentor but she is and always will be a true inspiration in how she has lived her life as a leader, philanthropist, and mother.

I strongly believe that emotional and mental well-being are the fundamentals of a healthy and happy life. But to understand resilience and compassion on a deeper level, I was fortunate to also study the Cognitively Based Compassion Training (CBCT) program at Emory University and went on to get teacher certification in 2020. I'm filled with gratitude to Professor Lobsang Tenzin Negi, Tim Harrison, and the CBCT teacher program for arming me with a road map of resilience and concepts that can be used in preventive mental health. Many of the tools that I discuss throughout my book are based on concepts from this course. Learning these principles has transformed my life, and it is my deep wish that these tools can help families in their lives as well.

The journey through medical school, residency, pediatrics, and authorship, along with the navigation of my life, has been a long and windy road and only possible because of the skills and tools I gained in my own childhood and the incredible support from my inner circle of care. My long and lazy summer visits to my loving Uncle Divakar's and Aunt Madhu's place as a kid meant being embraced and supported by a large family, which included my cousins, Nalin and Manjul; my sisters; and my grandparents, who would travel frequently from India to be with us. My grandfather, Dr P.L. Bhargava, was a professor and author of 19 books. He had a heart of gold and was a great influence on me, as was my grandma. My aunt, Mira, a mathematician and musician, was an incredible inspiration and taught me so much about persistence and the importance of goals. My loving dad, a statistician, taught me the lessons of hard work and dedication and appreciation of the simple gifts in life such as food and nature. And thank you to Sandeep, a wonderful father to our children. Finally, I would not be who I am today without the strong and constant influence of my mom, Shobhana. She is truly a hero and will always be my greatest inspiration. She raised me and my sisters as a single mom and never missed a parental beat. She is the strongest, smartest, and kindest person I know, and I will always strive to follow in her footsteps.

Last, but certainly not least, I'd like to express my deep gratitude to my circle of friends who have stood by me for years, through the good times and not so good. There are so many people who have stood unwavering by my side, but specifically I want to thank my sisters (yes, they are my best friends!), Dita and Aparna; their husbands; Ayala, an incredible mom, doctor, and dear friend of more than 30 years; and Peter and Fatima, amazing friends and doctors who have also been by my side for decades. I'd like to thank Meera and Chinmayee, 2 incredible sources of support in a time of crisis, as well as Renee, Beth, Miranda, Allyson, and Lynn. Each and every day, my sweet kids, Davik and Ellora, make me so happy and proud to be "Mom." This inner circle of friends and family have made me the parent, author, speaker, and doctor that I am today.

A close community or village is life's greatest gift, and for this I am, and will always be, eternally grateful.

I truly hope that after reading this book, the values and principles that have helped me and my children achieve resilience and contentment help you and your family "build happier" too.

Introduction

L

ife took on a force it of its own when my daughter was in fifth grade. Wake up, run, drive around, repeat. Days sped by fast, weeks even faster. We were on a merry-go-round that was spinning out of control. When my daughter was 10, she was involved in myriad activities. She was assigned a part in a play and was very excited about it. She also played in the town junior orchestra, requiring her to practice every night; she had basketball practice 3 times a week and games on Saturday. Eventually, basketball practice conflicted with play rehearsals. And, of course, homework was part of the mix, as the school prepared kids to transition to middle school. I often saw my daughter come home from drama or basketball by 8:00 pm, quickly eat and shower, and then do her homework. By the time she closed her eyes, it would be close to 10:30 pm.

Each day at 6:00 am, she would wake up and say, "I wish I could sleep in." As I thought about my upcoming workday, and my week's packed schedule, I didn't take this as seriously as I should have. I was exhausted juggling work, making meals, shopping for groceries, paying bills, doing laundry, and answering emails well into the evening, as was my spouse. We were both hanging on by a thread. Until the day my daughter woke up and announced that she wasn't going to school, that she just wanted to quit everything and stay in bed. I realized that my daughter's stress and anxiety had brought this on and she finally pulled the "Help!" alarm.

That finally made me stop in my tracks.

The Search for a "Perfect" Childhood

Questions formed in my mind that I couldn't answer. What was happening to my daughter? Why couldn't she handle it? Was it my fault? What happened to raising a grounded and balanced child who was armed with a robust toolbox to handle the challenges of life? Were we as parents and as a society driving our kids up the wall? I expect that a lot of parents have been in these shoes, exhausted and in pain, running on a hamster wheel with no end in sight.

As a pediatrician, I started asking around and heard similar stories from other parents about overscheduled, stressed-out kids. But in today's challenging world, children and teens are anxious for many other reasons as well, from national and global events; a pandemic; social issues; and concerns about health, safety, and climate change. Social media platforms can add to anxiety levels, depicting lives that look and seem better than yours. These concerns can be magnified by the 24/7 media barrage that brings news, social media, and online risks directly to our children on their smartphones, essentially providing a gateway to constant stress. Among the stories parents shared with me were of their children having panic attacks or depression, struggles at school, turning to vaping and drugs to self-medicate, and needing therapy or hospitalization for worsening mental health issues.

The patterns are undeniable—over the past few years, more children are anxious, stressed out, depressed, and even suicidal. Stress in a child is not rare; in fact, it is very common. Experts are reporting that 1 in 3 kids will develop anxiety by the time they are 18 years of age. Another factor that is less discussed, but should definitely be prioritized, is the stress that parents themselves feel on a day-to-day basis. Parents and caregivers are under more pressure than ever before. Economic challenges have forced some parents to take multiple jobs, leading to exhaustion and distancing themselves from their children. Other parents with resources may be yielding to family, culture, or societal pressure to raise high-achieving, successful "perfect" children, or they are trying to "keep up" with the idealized images they see on TV, movies, and digital media. What sometimes is forgotten is that parents' stress can often trigger children's stress as well.

Why is this happening to children and families now more than ever before? With hectic schedules, more academic and social demands, a lack of sleep, and an increase in screen use replacing face-to-face interactions, have kids *actually lost* what they need most—the protective layers that set them up for healthy growth and development? In the past, children were more engaged with their community, playing outside with neighborhood peers and chatting with their parents at the dinner table. Too much passively viewed TV is not good for anyone, but in the past, it didn't carry many of the risks of digital and social media that are present with today's computers and smartphones.

In the past, many of us believed that a "village" or community was present as a safety net to help us and our kids if needed. Do our kids know that such a community still exists for them? Do we as parents have access to the resources and support that can help us and our families in times of need? Now that life is busy and sometimes overwhelming for most families, we as parents seem to have less time to create, establish, and develop these protective layers. Many of us are juggling so much that we are in survival mode without a moment to step back and look at the big picture. Add a global crisis such as a pandemic with virtual learning and working from home to the family mix, and the alarm bells are clanging for almost everyone.

The Purpose of This Book

Clearly, life for parents and children has been growing more difficult. Stress was being caused by more than overscheduling, the digital media landscape, and economic and social pressures. In my position as a medical editor and director at WebMD, I was fortunate to be able to access the latest research on children and adolescents and stress. I started researching the increased levels of stress, their causes, and options for prevention and treatment. I also was able to take a teacher certification in Cognitive Based Compassion Training at Emory University, which taught me principles in emotional and mental well-being.

I decided to write this book, because, as a pediatrician (and mother!) I am worried that the constant pressures of our society have led us to lose sight of the basic building blocks to form the foundation of healthy adulthood. Children and teens need a life toolbox that can provide them with the tools and skills to face challenges and be successful and happy. As a parent of twin teens, I have struggled to unplug from the daily "runaway train," and, instead of focusing on what our plugged-in society or even I might want for my children, focus on who my children are and what they want and need. Making a change requires a pause for reflection—stopping the treadmill and scheduling the basics, while removing things that do not serve our family's mental and physical well-being.

The perfect storm of schedules, screens, social media, sleeplessness, and society have led to our stressed-out children whose emotional and mental health has suffered. We are faced with the modern digital media environment at every turn. But many of us are unsure about what to do about the increased smartphone and tablet use that seeps into almost every moment of our families' lives. As we all struggle to manage time, we have sacrificed the basics, which include the 4 pillars—sleep, nutrition, downtime, and healthy relationships. These pillars can mitigate stress and lay a healthy foundation for children to be happier now *and* in the future.

I recently pulled my son out of tennis so that he could focus on a standardized test that was coming up; we took a break from my daughter's orchestra practice so she could have a few days to just rest and reset. We have started thinking carefully about attending social events, parties, and sleepovers as opposed to sharing downtime at home together to just "veg." We have started practicing meditation and deep breathing exercises. And I, personally, have carved out time to use my stationary bike or lift weights even if it's just for 30 minutes. As hard as it may be to find these small moments, it's important that parents prioritize their own health so they can better promote the health of their children. To make a change, we need to take a pause and reconsider many decisions.

When I started pulling my kids from certain activities, or pausing others, to make time for them to recover and reset, and for us as a family to see the bigger picture, my children initially resisted. But most children are adaptable, with elastic minds. Once my children realized how reevaluating and resetting life's values and obligations made us all feel better, they embraced the changes. And when I started taking time to go for a run or enjoy coffee with a friend, I was in a much better place as a parent to communicate calmly with my kids and address their questions and concerns. With our reset, we saw differences in our ability to handle stress quickly. We became much more flexible in our thinking, a tool which promotes resiliency.

In this book, I outline the essential buffers and basics that can protect our kids (and ourselves!) from being pulled into a daily grind that can have serious negative consequences on our kids' health of our kids. I discuss common issues, talk about relevant cases, and provide short quizzes to help you identify concerns that stress your family. Most importantly, I offer toolbox takeaways to help you make small, doable changes that can have the most beneficial effect. Change for the better will take some work and some time, but at the end of the day, your children will build a toolbox of lifelong skills they need to be healthy physically, mentally, and emotionally. I look forward to working with you all on that exciting journey!

How Strong Is Your Child's Emotional Well-being?

1. How often does your child seem worried or complain of stomachaches or headaches?*
    a. Daily (5 points)
    b. A few times a week (4 points)
    c. Once or twice a week (3 points)
    d. Once or twice a month (2 points)
    e. Almost never (1 point)

2. Does your child ever have trouble making decisions?
    a. Yes, most of the time (5 points)
    b. Occasionally (3 points)
    c. Almost never (1 point)

3. How often does your child connect with friends they know either online or in person?
    a. Almost never (5 points)
    b. Occasionally (3 points)
    c. Pretty much all the time (1 point)

*Although headaches and stomachaches can be a sign of stress, they can also be a sign of physical illness. If your child frequently has headaches or stomachaches, talk to your pediatrician.

4. When your child makes a mistake or experiences a setback, do they bounce back quickly?

    a. Almost never—they are usually devastated, and it takes a long time for them to recover. (5 points)

    b. Sometimes—it might take them a few days, but they are usually back on their feet within a week or less. (3 points)

    c. Pretty much always—my child doesn't dwell much on mistakes or failures. (1 point)

5. How would you describe your relationship with your child?

    a. It's nonexistent; we have trouble connecting most of the time. (5 points)

    b. We have our ups and downs, and probably more downs than ups. (4 points)

    c. We have trouble understanding each other at times, but our relationship is mostly solid. (2 points)

    d. We communicate honestly with each other and usually spend at least a little time talking together every day. (1 point)

Add up your score. Total _____

What Your Score Means

0 to 5 points: Yes! Your child seems to have some decent strategies for coping with anxiety. It's important to keep the conversation between the 2 of you going so you can ensure that they're continuing to do well and you can spot any problems before they grow more severe.

6 to 15 points: You and your child are doing some things well to manage your child's mental health, but it's important to keep mental and emotional well-being a priority through tools such as communication and community. Make an effort to see your child one-on-one at least once a day at a regular time so that they know they can talk with you if they need to.

16 to 25 points: Strong mental health is a key for a child to thrive. You and your child may need to adopt more strategies that promote mental well-being, and we'll explore many possibilities in this chapter. If you have any concerns about your kid's mental health, talk to your pediatrician for a referral to a mental health care practitioner. (But act quickly if your child signals that they're suicidal. To learn more about the signs of a problem, see Chapter 8.)

CHAPTER 1

Building Your Mental Health Toolbox

As a pediatrician, I've talked with a lot of parents and heard how much they desire the best for their children, as well as the pressure they feel to ensure their children are emotionally, mentally, and physically healthy. I've heard and seen the effect of this constant stress on each part of their families' lives. They've shared with me the hours spent driving their children back and forth to sports, to play practices, and to school events such as choir concerts and drama productions. From some parents, I heard about test preparation, writing coaches, and college tours and the extra time and effort parents spent helping their kids apply to colleges. Most parents have shared their concerns about their children spending too much time on their phones or computers, and fears about keeping them safe online. As a mom of 2 teenagers myself, I've experienced plenty of this worry and stress firsthand. In this book, we take a close look at the factors that can contribute to increased stress, such as overscheduling, lack of sleep, and excessive digital media use, and how in the quest to make our children happier and healthier, we've often compromised the fundamentals that can make a big difference in their lives. I'm excited to share these great ideas and tips and tools to ensure these fundamentals remain an important part of your and your family's overall happiness and well-being.

Mental health is vital for children to feel content and be able to cope in the face of adversity. But what happens when mental and emotional well-being become compromised? Anxiety in kids has been on the rise, as has depression. A 2018 study showed that the incidence of anxiety in teens increased by 20%, and one-third of kids between the ages of 13 and 18 will have an anxiety disorder diagnosed. Stress can often increase in college. This was evident in a 2018 study where nearly 41% of college students reported feeling "overwhelming anxiety."

The state of your child's mental health can affect their physical health as well. Children and teens with a history of anxiety and depression are more likely to develop irritable bowel syndrome, endure asthma attacks, or experience migraines. Anxiety can interfere with quality sleep and the fundamentals for good health such as good nutrition and proper exercise. Additionally, anxiety or depression can muddy thinking; people in a low or anxious state often have trouble making decisions and seeing things clearly. These feelings may be consistent and can be distracting for children, making it difficult to focus on studying, perform well on a test, or listen closely to a parent or friend. I think of anxiety or a low mood as a state similar to wearing smudged-up glasses: these emotions make it difficult for children to see the world with clarity and to function well. The question is this: How can we keep the lenses clear so our children can thrive? Are there tools we can learn to help our children manage everyday stressors?

Allow Your Children to Learn Resilience

Some experts have indicated that "helicoptering" our kids may contribute to anxiety. Not only are our kids running around with their plates too full, but we as parents oversee every aspect of their lives. Are we raising children who don't have the proper skills to cope with life's everyday challenges because we remove every obstacle in their path? How might this affect their resilience and ability to pivot in difficult or challenging situations?

Melanie, a 16-year-old, has parents who are highly educated working professionals who would do anything for her. For prom, Melanie's mother bought her a dress and 3 different types of shoes because Melanie couldn't decide which she liked best. If there was a problem with a teacher or Melanie's academic performance, her parents immediately swooped in to fix the situation by arranging a conference or hiring a tutor. Despite her parents' heavy involvement in mitigating many high-pressure situations, Melanie was anxious and often seemed to be stressed out about everything. Her family is not alone in this dynamic. One study of more than 3,600 parents showed that no matter the economic or cultural background, many parents spent increasing amounts of time and energy on parenting and barely left their child's side. Other research revealed that time-intensive parenting leads to kids feeling less confident in their own abilities and more likely to experience anxiety and stress.

It's natural to want to protect our children; this instinct is encoded in our DNA. But when we clear their pathway of any obstacles, we eliminate opportunities for our children to learn how to pick themselves up when they fall. We cheat them out of the chance to practice critical thinking skills in new situations and allow them to manage and work through challenges on their own. Given our hectic schedules, it's not uncommon to lack the time to allow kids to experiment, to try and possibly fail.

It is often difficult as a parent not to go in and just "fix everything." But sometimes, that's not necessarily what your child wants to hear. When my son was in eighth grade, he shared with me how overwhelmed he felt with the amount of homework he received daily. After listening to his concerns, I immediately jumped in and starting firing away questions about what was due, when was it due, how much he had completed, and so forth. I was surprised when he yelled that I didn't understand and that I always made him feel like he wasn't good enough. After a bit of reflection, I realized that my son had wanted me simply to *listen* while he unloaded and vented his stress. In my hurry to jump in and help fix the problem, I didn't focus on what my son initially needed, and that was to be a supportive sounding board. Listening to how a person feels can sometimes be cathartic for the stressed-out person. By listening (and not responding quickly), you provide yourself a chance to notice if that person is merely venting or is seeking out advice or assistance from you. After that person has shared their concerns or fears with you, it is useful to acknowledge out loud what they are feeling. "I hear that you are struggling with your workload after school. I am sorry you are stressed out. What are some ways you think you might be able to manage this?" This lets your child know you have listened to everything they have said and gives them a chance to figure out a solution on their own with you as a supportive guide.

Preserving the Parent-Child Relationship

It's important to understand how important your role is in your child's life and that your choices as a parent can influence the connection you build with your child. At times, you may serve as a buffer to shield them from *too much* stress. When it came to my friend Magda and her son Matty, who was a senior in high school, she spent most of the fall reminding him about his college essays and other application materials. Matty was a bright student, and his parents were optimistic about his promising college career ahead. But as the weeks passed and Matty avoided completing his applications, Magda's anxiety and frustration mounted. Multiple family dinners ended in a lot of yelling and heated arguments.

The family visited a therapist who helped them talk through their ongoing situation, addressing why Matty was dragging his feet with college applications. The arguments were no longer about the applications but had become a power struggle. The therapist praised Magda and Matty for their close connection and suggested that the dinner table be a safe space for family conversations reserved only for eating, unwinding, and connecting with one another and no stress-inducing discussions. This pause avoided battles and allowed Matty to see the situation more clearly. Stressful topics could be addressed at other times and could even be scheduled for a time when all family members were prepared to share. This simple change safeguarded their family time and helped strengthen their communication. It allowed them all to choose a better time to discuss Matty's plans for after high school and move forward with a plan the entire family was on board with.

ADAPTING TO A NEW NORMAL

The pandemic of 2020 put kids' (and parents') mental and emotional well-being to the test. As it became clear that the pandemic would continue, graduation season became a source of disappointment and stress for many kids and teens. They not only missed out on graduations and summer parties but graduating high school seniors also faced universities and colleges not reopening in the fall. These unexpected changes required tools that we all need: *resilience* and *adaptability*. For many kids and teens, this was their first significant encounter with adversity and the unexpected events that life can throw at us. In such situations, the ability to pivot and to think outside the box both help. Kids figured out ways to socialize virtually or by going out for walks with masks on. They spent more time at home on activities they enjoyed such as board games, puzzles, and baking. They realized the silver lining of not having the rush of activities—more time with each other and more time to reset. These skills became even more important as the world awaited a vaccine and many schools held classes virtually.

Parents can encourage their child's adaptability by celebrating the moments when they brainstorm alternatives and embrace a plan B. We as parents also can model the skill of moving beyond our own disappointment to find silver linings.

I loved the creative pivot approach of one family at graduation time. When the combo graduation and 18th birthday party the family had envisioned for their son was canceled, they still celebrated by inviting family and friends to drive by in decorated cars for a funny graduation parade. Their son greeted them all in his front yard wearing his cap and gown and danced to music from speakers on the porch. Even though this celebration looked and felt different and could not ease all his disappointment, his mom was proud and praised him for adapting to the changes.

Mental Illness in Children

I've often had concerned parents ask me if their child's behavior might signal a *mental illness*, which is defined as any changes in thinking, feeling, or behaving that cause distress or disrupt someone's ability to function. An estimated 1 in 5 kids has a mental illness, and signs pointing to one can worry parents significantly, especially as coverage in the media displays disturbing news that a growing number of kids have anxiety and other mental disorders. Some conditions can be inherited, similar to the way a physical disease can.

Some common mental illnesses in children include the following:

- **Anxiety disorders.** These involve persistent fears or worries that can affect your child's performance at school or their level of enjoyment in extracurricular activities. They include generalized anxiety disorder, obsessive compulsive disorder, and social anxiety.
- **Eating disorders.** Children or teens with an eating disorder are often preoccupied with the appearance of their body, have a distorted view of their weight, and have unhealthy eating habits. Common eating disorders include anorexia nervosa and bulimia.
- **Depressive disorders.** Depression involves persistent feelings of sadness and loss of interest in activities that your child once enjoyed. In some cases, depression can be a symptom of bipolar disorder, which involves an emotional pendulum swinging their mood between extreme lows and extreme highs.

The following are possible situations your child may experience that can be attributed to mental disorder symptoms:

- A low mood that lasts for 2 or more weeks
- Avoiding friends and social interactions
- A loss of interest in activities your child used to enjoy
- Hurting their body or talking about hurting themselves
- Talking about death or suicide
- A change in eating habits, loss of appetite, or significant weight loss or gain
- Sudden aggressive outbursts or extreme irritability
- Sleeping excessively or difficulty sleeping
- Frequent headaches or stomachaches
- A sudden, unexpected decline in grades

Do not wait or dismiss these statements as child or teenage drama. If you suspect that your child is contemplating harming themselves or is following through on self-harm, or has alluded to suicide or suicidal thoughts such as saying, "Nothing matters," or "I wonder how many people would come to my funeral?" reach out for help from a mental health care practitioner *immediately*. If you have questions about finding a practitioner, one option is to call the National Suicide Prevention Lifeline at 800/273-8255.

PARENTAL SELF-CARE

Self-care and replenishment are essential tools to be at our best as a parent. Do we take time to ground ourselves? Reports have recently shown that parental stress is at an all-time high and that that is because many of us have forgotten that we cannot continue to give without replenishment. Think about the oxygen mask when you take a flight. We are asked to put on the oxygen mask *first*, before putting it on our children. Similarly, if we don't do this in real life, we ourselves can reach a point of burnout and therefore won't be able to give all that we need to our children. See Chapter 7 for strategies on managing parental stress and refilling your cup.

Tools to Strengthen Our Children's Mental Health

Research suggests that children can experience a form of social isolation when they're glued to their digital devices, particularly if they're scrolling endlessly on social media, which offers a host of emotional pitfalls for vulnerable teens. Although technologies such as online meetings and video games can be valuable platforms to connect, not all virtual connections are equally useful and sustaining for our families. No digital device or online platform can replace face-to-face interaction. We know the constant 24/7 news cycle—including the alarming headlines that appear on digital devices every time a crisis unfolds—may only exacerbate anxiety and stress for a child of any age. Many parents worry about how social and digital media can affect their children's mental health, and the possible long-term effects these can have, which we'll examine on a deeper level in Chapter 4.

When practiced regularly, the following tools can help strengthen your child's ability to feel calm, grounded, and secure and adapt to challenges when they arise. I encourage you to read through each of these tools and start with 1 or 2 that may resonate with your family. You may find yourself adopting 1 or more of these strategies that can serve your family well into the future.

Tool 1: Parent-Child Connection

Action: Foster a strong connection with your child and teen.

How to Implement: A strong connection can build a sense of security; nurturing builds a sense of self-efficacy, allowing kids to have the confidence to explore different environments. Research has shown that the single most important factor in helping a child develop resilience is a strong and nurturing relationship with an adult. Children do best when they know that a parent or caregiver loves them uncondi-tionally and believes in them. When they feel secure in at least 1 relationship, kids can thrive, even when faced with adverse life experiences, such as long-term sickness, the divorce of their parents, or death of a loved one. It is import-ant to nurture the parent-child bond, prioritize family time, and make choices that foster healthy communication.

One family I know went through a tough divorce. The parents were at odds for several years, and the father left the home in a trial separation. It was a painful time, but the mother made it a priority to schedule regular one-on-one time alone with each of her children. It was through these moments that she was able to continue fostering and build-ing confidence within each of her children and strengthen-ing their emotional centers so they could continue to thrive.

Be physically and emotionally present. Check in regularly with younger children at the dinner table or when you tuck them into bed. Be sure to make time for your older children as well, even if they don't seem to want it. Consistency matters; making it a habit to talk with your children on most days gives them regular opportunities to share their thoughts, worries, concerns, or even a laugh, when and if they need to talk. Listen-ing often and keeping an ear close to what your children say to you can give you insight into what they may be worried about or what they are thinking—and can help you step in if needed. Taking the time to invest in your children's emotional well-be-ing helps build and sustain a positive, healthy relationship that will thrive through the teenage years and into adulthood.

Tool 2: Building Resilience Skills

Action: Help your kids embrace missteps.

How to Implement: Kids will inevitably experience a range of challenges in life, and it's beneficial for them to know that even when they make a big mistake or stumble, a solution can always be found. We often think that raising successful, happy children is making sure they achieve performance victories such as an A in algebra, a flawless performance in a school play, or the winning goal during a soccer game. But success is best achieved when we sometimes allow our children to stumble and pick themselves up. An unsatisfying performance is an opportunity for your child to learn the importance of additional practice or an indication that they need strategies to deal with stage fright and learn ways to relax their nerves and have fun!

For some kids, it helps to learn the stories of great athletes who might seem like they were born perfect. But their journeys show that the climb to the top involved failing—a lot—and learning how to keep moving forward after those failures. The legendary basketball player Michael Jordan explained that mistakes were part of building his skills. "I've missed more than 9,000 shots in my career," he once said. "I've lost almost 300 games. Twenty-six times, I've been trusted to take the game-winning shot and missed. I've failed over and over and over again in my life. And that is why I succeed."

At home, I often talk about how mistakes are part of life and usually are important learning opportunities. Always praise your child on the effort they did put into the test or recital, even if they made a mistake or had a less-than-stellar performance. And if your child fails a test or flubs an audition, give them time to process those feelings of disappointment. When they are ready, suggest that they brainstorm ways to perform better next time. Share stories of your own struggles, a fight with a friend, a project at work that went south, or the death of a loved one. Talk about how you faced these events, including what went well and what didn't help and what you learned from the experiences.

Tool 3: A Sense of Safety

Action: Help your children regain a sense of safety.

How to Implement: Although in most cases the word *grounding* is associated with punishment, it is also referred to as a technique that can help a child regain a sense of safety. This technique is very helpful in stressful situations. When a person is stressed or feeling out of control, the person begins noticing the places where the body is currently making direct contact with a surface. The idea is to scan the body mentally, paying close attention to the places where the body is being supported.

When your child is feeling anxious or worried or is experiencing strong emotions, sit them down and have them notice the way the floor supports their feet, how their toes touch the insides of their shoes, or how the couch cushions are snug against their back. They might notice how their legs press against the couch and the way their hands rest on their lap. The idea is to boost their awareness of the support provided by their surroundings and to shift their attention away from the negative or anxious feelings to focus on neutral or pleasant sensations. It's a calming mindfulness technique that is a little simpler and easier than meditation for some children and teens to practice. In fact, this technique has been used for adults who are frontline health care workers by the Trauma Resource Institute and is incorporated into the Community Resiliency Model. In several studies, this was found to decrease anxiety for working nurses or emergency medical technicians. Practice grounding a few times with your child, and then suggest that they use the technique in other circumstances: at their desk at school a few minutes before taking a test, outside during lunch or recess, or sitting on the school bus.

Tool 4: Resourcing

Action: Help your child/teen reflect on their favorite experiences.

How to Implement: Another helpful technique, known as *resourcing*, involves recalling a person, place, animal, or other memory that evokes a sense of well-being for your child. This can be a great conversation starter with your child before bed. Ask them to describe a specific time when they felt content and at ease, and encourage them to fill in the memory with as many sensory details as possible. For example, if they're recalling the first time they met the family dog, they might remember how his fuzzy ears felt under their fingertips, the smell of his fur, the sound of his little puppy bark. Encourage them to create a short, 30-second mental memory of this experience that they can replay in their mind in situations when they're feeling anxious or panicky. As a parent, you might consider creating your own mental memory reel and use this tool in stressful circumstances, such as before a high-pressure business meeting.

Each of us strives to reconnect with ourselves in order to feel our best. We look for moments when we're in a place to feel balanced mentally and physically. Most of us have experienced moments or even days when we feel able to handle challenges and find solutions. Some mental health care practitioners call those moments the "Resilient Zone," and techniques such as resourcing and grounding can help us enter that zone or return to it when stressful experiences become overwhelming. Talking about the Resilient Zone with your kids can be useful because it gives you language to discuss mental and emotional states and the best ways each of you can reach the zone.

Tool 5: Independence and Decision-making Practice

Action: Assign new responsibilities to your kids.

How to Implement: Teens crave independence, and when they have the ability to make decisions on their own, they develop an important skill known as *self-efficacy*. This is a person's belief in their own abilities, especially the power to handle challenges when they arise. But because our kids' lives are so scheduled, with very little unstructured time, it can often create increased amounts of stress that can make it more difficult for children or teens to practice critical-thinking skills or decision-making. In some cases, these high-pressure situations can lead to self-doubt and lack of confidence in their decision-making skills.

So how can we help our children build these independent thinking skills and strengthen their confidence? One mother shared with me that her 11-year-old daughter, Reilly, was assigned certain chores at home. Starting at age 9, Reilly was in charge of her own laundry. The first few weeks after being assigned her new responsibilities, Reilly forgot to do her laundry and ran out of clothes. Instead of fixing the problem by doing laundry for her, Reilly's mother gave Reilly the opportunity to realize she still had to follow through on her responsibility, even if she forgot. Some parents might view this approach as harsh, but Reilly's mother viewed it as a way to encourage her daughter to develop important skills such as accountability. Over time, Reilly figured out a routine for her chores and doing laundry.

LESSONS LEARNED FROM PARENTING THROUGH A PANDEMIC

During the height of the pandemic in 2020, parents were stretched beyond belief. Working parents found themselves having to manage online schooling with older children or figuring out child care for their younger kids at home. During these times, parents shared with me that they were stressed and looking for answers on how best to navigate this unprecedented time. The following are tools I discussed with each of these families:

- **Focus on what is important at that moment.** Let go of what isn't. Is it more important that the house is clean or that a proper breakfast or lunch is offered to your children? We are human and cannot do everything at once. It should not all be left up to the parents. Once the important, urgent needs are met, work with your family members to make sure everyone is stepping up and contributing something within the household. Children can help clean up their toys while dinner is being made. Your teenager can safely take out the dog while you attend to bath time with the younger siblings. Letting go of things and delegating chores when possible can help you focus on what's most important, allowing you to get done what is needed and avoid excessive stress.

- **Lean into your adult relationships.** When stress is in overdrive, the sympathetic system of our body (fight-or-flight response) is triggered. To balance this, we need our parasympathetic system, which is activated by calming actions such as talking to a friend, receiving a hug, or breathing more slowly and deeply. Taking time to connect with another human being virtually, spending time with a spouse, or going on a (COVID safe!) walk with a friend can also help during stressful times.

- **Look for silver linings.** It comes as no surprise that many people struggled during the pandemic and may still be struggling. One silver lining that many families learned to embrace was the availability of time. More time spent at home meant more time spent with family on interactive activities such as puzzles, board games, and arts and crafts. The usual rush of running from 1 activity to the other was gone and allowed more time for parents to engage with their children. At home, my children and I found ourselves baking quite a bit, playing board games, and watching old TV shows.

Tool 6: Community

Action: Teach your child the importance of people they can count on.

How to Implement: You and your spouse and the other caregivers in your family will always play important roles in your child's life. As human beings, we are social creatures, made to be connected to others. We crave a sense of belonging, of knowing that we are part of something larger than ourselves. We all need to feel supported and loved, and community is a particularly important component of wellness for children, who are reassured when they know they have a "village" of people ready and willing to help them.

Community comes in many forms. It can be the place of worship your family attends; the extended family of cousins, uncles, aunts, and grandparents; the neighbors; families you meet at your child's school; or the teammates on your child's soccer team. A supportive community is any group of people that knows you and your child by name. Your community can also provide your children and teens with myriad trusted adults who they can turn to outside of their parents. This might include an aunt, coach, religious leader, teacher, therapist, or other adult whom your teen respects and with whom they feel comfortable sharing their thoughts and ideas. This is especially important as children work to develop independence. During the times when your child seems to resist everything you say, it can feel helpful to know that they have someone to turn to who is supportive. This is a great conversation starter to pursue with your child at dinner or before bed. Ask them, "Who are the safe adults you can talk to if I'm not available?" Make sure they have that person's phone number or email for those times when they're ready to connect.

Tool 7: The Circles of Action

Action: Help your child or teen to accept what is in their control—and what's not.

How to Implement: The Circles of Action is a diagram that can ease a child's anxiety by helping them think about what they can truly control in life (including their own words and actions) and encouraging them to let go of what they cannot control or act upon (Figure 1.1). It might be helpful to print out or sketch a version of these circles to hang on the fridge or bathroom mirror for your child to remind them as they go about their daily routines. A child who experiences high stress and anxiety over making the school track team or applying to a specific college may feel less anxious if they are confident they practiced and prepared to the best of their ability, realizing that the decision of making the team or being accepted into the college is out of their hands. Regardless of the outcome, whether positive or disappointing, they can still lean back on the fact they did the best they could with the resources they had.

FIGURE 1.1
Circles of Action

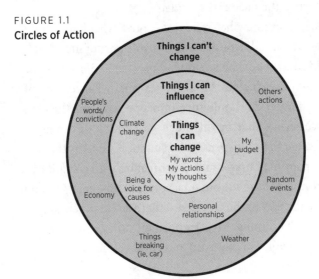

The Circles of Action can also provide you the opportunity to talk with your child about perspective and how they choose to respond to or view negative experiences. Buddhist teachers often explore this idea with the story of the old farmer whose horse ran away. His neighbors came to visit and shook their heads, saying, "Such bad luck."

"Maybe," the farmer responded.

The next day, the horse came back to the farmer's barn, bringing 3 wild horses with him. The neighbors responded with excitement. "Such good luck!" they said.

"Maybe," the farmer responded.

The next day, the farmer's son rode 1 of the new wild horses and it threw him off, breaking his leg. "Such bad luck," the neighbors lamented.

"Maybe," the farmer responded.

The next morning, soldiers came to the village to draft young men for war but seeing that the farmer's son had a broken leg, they passed him by. "Wow, such good luck!" the neighbors exclaimed.

"Maybe," the farmer responded.

The farmer knew he could not control what happened to him—ups and downs are an inevitable part of life—but he *could* control how he responded or what actions he took regarding those changes. He also knew that what seemed like a bad outcome 1 day could turn into a positive one the next (and vice versa). Sharing this story with your kids can help them change their perspective on situations. Events that feel brutally painful at first—such as a breakup with a significant other or not making the cut on a sports team—may turn out not to be the end of the world and there could potentially even be a silver lining. Most importantly, they can choose how they respond to that pain and choose whether acting on it makes sense.

Making Mental Health a Priority for Kids

A healthy state of mind can make a huge difference in a child's life, so it's important to do what we can as parents and role models to ensure that our children are safe, happy, and healthy. For some of us, a lot of focus has been placed on ensuring that kids are academically successful and accepted into elite colleges, while for others it's been tremendous pressure for kids to succeed in athletics. Both of these often point to to the fact that kids' and teens' mental well-being has fallen to the wayside. Although school, sports, and achievement are important, there are other priorities as well that cannot be compromised and can lead to mental health issues, anxiety, increased stress, or depression. Many schools are now including social and emotional learning into the curriculum. It's important for parents to ensure that if their child has a mental health condition they're receiving quality care from a mental health care practitioner and that their child continues to receive mental health care for as long as needed. Reflect on what your children are learning about mental health and well-being by observing you every day, with you as their guiding light.

Toolbox Takeaways for Mental Health

TAKEAWAY 1: **Laughter**

Nothing resets a bad mood or reconnects you with your child or teen faster than sharing a sincere, whole-body laugh. When you find a funny online video, book, or meme, share it with your family. Find out what makes your child roll on the floor laughing. Make dates to watch laugh-out-loud movies and TV shows together, even if it's only once a week. In time, you may find your child looking forward to these scheduled days.

TAKEAWAY 2: Safety

Establish a code word that your kids can give you when they need you to remove them from an unsafe or uncomfortable situation, no questions asked. This should be something a child feels comfortable putting into action at any hour of any day. This may prevent them from making risky choices, avoid judgment, and help cement your level of trust and connection to each other.

TAKEAWAY 3: Emotions

Post a dry-erase board in the kitchen. Ask each family member to rank how they're feeling on a scale of 1 to 10 (1 feeling low and 10 feeling happy) and write their number on the board daily. It's especially helpful for children and teens who have trouble putting feelings into words and provides you a topic to chat about before bed.

TAKEAWAY 4: Dance

Give all family members permission to declare whole-family dance breaks. Blast an infectious song and commit to going nutty until the song ends. This will raise your heart rate and mood in just minutes. If your teen rolls their eyes, see if they have a favorite song they are willing to sing out loud with you. Singing together can also lift your moods!

TAKEAWAY 5: Hugs

Give all members of the family a hug anytime. Hugging can help release oxytocin, a hormone that calms us and makes us feel better. If your child or teen is grumpy or upset, ask if it's OK to give them a hug. And don't be afraid to ask for one yourself, too.

QUIZ

Is Your Family Embracing the Basics?

1. How often does your child eat vegetables or fruit?
   - a. With every meal (0 points)
   - b. Once or twice a day (1 point)
   - c. Several times a week (3 points)
   - d. About once a week (4 points)
   - e. Almost never (5 points)

2. How many times per week does your child eat sugary foods?
   - a. Never (0 points)
   - b. Maybe once or twice (1 point)
   - c. 2 or 3 times (2 points)
   - d. 4 or 5 times (3 points)
   - e. Probably every day (4 points)
   - f. Every day, multiple times a day (5 points)

3. How many glasses of water does your child typically drink in 1 day?
- a. 6 to 8 glasses (0 points)
- b. 4 or 5 glasses (1 point)
- c. 2 or 3 glasses (2 points)
- d. 1 or 2 glasses (4 points)
- e. None (5 points)

4. How many days per week does your child get 9 to 10 hours of uninterrupted sleep?
- a. 7 days (0 points)
- b. 6 days (1 point)
- c. 4 or 5 days (2 points)
- d. 2 or 3 days (3 points)
- e. Maybe once (4 points)
- f. Never (5 points)

5. How many days per week does your child engage in at least an hour of physical activity?
- a. Every day (0 points)
- b. 5 or 6 days (1 point)
- c. 3 or 4 days (2 points)
- d. 1 or 2 days (3 points)
- e. None (5 points)

Add up your score. Total _____

What Your Score Means

0 to 8 points: Congrats! Your family has an impressive handle on the fundamentals of a healthy lifestyle. A strong foundation of sleep, a wholesome diet, plenty of water, and a commitment to being active will serve your kids (and you!) well in life. This chapter offers many ideas to build on these successes and keep your family on track, even during times when your schedule is extra hectic.

9 to 16 points: The good news—your family has some terrific healthy habits. But a few small changes in your routine can really transform life for your kids—and you. The advice in this chapter offers a lot of tips to address the pillars of good health and fortify your family for daily life.

17 to 25 points: Your family sounds as though it might be struggling with the basics. Take a look at this chapter and review the many ideas on ways that you can nudge you and your children toward healthier habits. Let's get started!

CHAPTER 2

Finding Your Way Back to the 4 Fundamentals

As a parent with a busy life, do you ever wonder what the magic solution to success and happiness is? Do you ever wonder how other families manage the stressors in their life? Is there a simple strategy that will affect every aspect of your child's life positively and make sure they are healthy and strong? Is there a one-stop, overall answer to staying happy?

The problem is that as we try to do it all, we struggle to manage it, and in the end, we often lose the fundamentals, and sacrifice our own happiness. Doing it all, we realize, is not as simple as we thought. Whether it's joining the baseball travel team or ensuring our kids volunteer outside of school in order to add those activities to college applications, or keeping up with our friends, it can be easy to lose sight of the 4 basic foundation pillars that are beneficial and vital to a family's health and happiness. For some families, healthy routines become more difficult to maintain when life is disrupted or during times of high pressure or stress. But it is during these particular moments when the basics become even more important to help our kids stay strong, healthy, and resilient.

WORKING WITH ANXIETY

At 13, Ella seemed to be doing well for herself. She received straight A's, was on the honor roll, played cello for the city orchestra, and was on a neighborhood tennis team. She was very bright and seemed pretty content. All of that changed the day she had a panic attack on the tennis court. After losing a match, she sat on the bench and began having trouble breathing. Worried about her daughter having an asthma attack, her mother rushed her to the hospital. While talking to her, the doctor listened as Ella explained her anxiety: often coming home late after tennis practice, staying up all hours of the night completing homework, getting up early to see her teacher for extra math help, cello practice, and playing tennis. When asked about meals, Ella indicated she ate cereal but sometimes forgot to take snacks for in between her tennis matches.

It may not surprise anyone why Ella experienced high anxiety: lack of sleep, missed nutrition and hydration, and plenty of stress. The doctor discussed the effect of each of these with Ella and her mother so that Ella could start making smarter, healthier decisions moving forward. Not getting enough sleep, food, or even water could certainly make her more likely to experience this type of episode. One recommendation was for her to remove an activity or 2 from her schedule so she could focus on the other activities and be more present with those efforts. The doctor also recommended that if Ella's anxiety increased, to consider talking with a therapist once her schedule became manageable.

Fundamental 1—The Right Foods

As kids get older, they often become pickier, especially about making healthy food choices such as vegetables. Choosing to make healthy, nutritious food as part of daily meals is vital to brain development, growth, and emotional well-being.

Vitamins, minerals, and antioxidants are found in fresh fruit and vegetables, as well as in legumes. Vitamin C, vitamin E, and beta-carotene, along with minerals such as zinc, can help fight and prevent diseases such as heart disease and cancer. Many parents often wonder if a vitamin supplement can be used instead of constantly encouraging children to eat more fruits and veggies. Although over-the-counter vitamins can be somewhat helpful, those don't match up to the real food; they may be missing an essential nutritional component (such as polyphenols in strawberries) that are important to fight disease, and there are questions about whether they are absorbed by the body in the same way as nutrients in real food. Real foods also play such an important role in making sure our immune system is armed and ready for infections that we may encounter.

Figure 2.1 illustrates the 5 key components that make up a healthy meal. It is a general guide for nutrition and what your plate should look like for daily meals. As indicated, half of the plate should be fruits and vegetables. There are more specific guidelines available online, but this is a useful starting point to explain food group proportions.

FIGURE 2.1
US Department of Agriculture MyPlate—How to Build a Healthy Plate

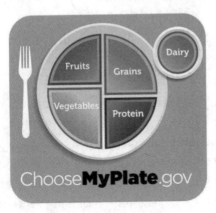

Source: https://www.choosemyplate.gov/resources/myplate-graphic-resources

Triple Threat: Salt, Sugar, and Processed Foods

Our goals as parents are well intentioned—we *want* to feed our kids healthy food. But juggling a fast-paced life can make it challenging, and an easy fix is to grab and go instead of cooking.

Salt

It's probably no surprise that many drive-through fast-food options contain ingredients that are unhealthy. Because salty foods taste good, most restaurant foods offer the following:

- Food that contains at least 30% more salt than home-cooked meals
- Foods with empty calories
- Foods with a lot of added preservatives and chemicals
- Food packaging in plastic or coated paper that may contain toxins that could be endocrine disruptors
- Portion sizes greater than what you might serve at home

Fast foods are not the only types that promote unhealthy options. Even certain foods found in the grocery store not only lack nutrients but also are calorie and salt heavy.

Food Quiz: Which food contains the most salt?

> a. Smoked chipotle chicken
> b. Frozen pizza
> c. Whole wheat bread
> d. Canned black beans

While types of food and brands vary in sodium content, all of these foods are high in sodium levels. And we are all victims of too much salt consumption—the average person eats about 5 or more teaspoons of salt a day. Although our bodies need salt, too much can cause fluid imbalance in our bodies and set us up for chronic health problems such as high blood pressure. Most people need only 1,500 mg of salt a day;

children need even less. But the good news is that once you start reducing your salt intake, you will become accustomed to it, and your salt cravings will subside.

The following are some general ways to avoid excessive salt intake:

- Decrease the amount of purchased pizza, cured meats, and canned foods.
- Look at the percentage of salt on nutrition labels; a single meal should include no more than 20% of your daily salt intake (see Figure 2.1).
- Limit the number of times you order in or go out.
- Plan meals ahead of time; ask your family members to help you choose fun recipes to make.

THE DOWNSIDE TO PLASTICS: PHTHALATES

One of the common chemicals that we should be aware of is a class known as *phthalates.* Phthalates are human-made chemicals that can affect the endocrine system and are known as *endocrine disruptors.* These chemicals are added to plastic products to make them more flexible but can also be found in personal care products such as lotions, cosmetics, and fragrances. Phthalates are often found in plastic wrapping and even wrappers that are used in fast-food restaurants. One study that looked at more than 10,000 people found that there were increased levels of phthalates in their urine the day after eating out. The study's authors concluded that 1 way to reduce exposure would be to eat at home more, paying attention to foods that are not wrapped in plastic and reducing foods that are canned. Lastly, there is more evidence that toxins can contribute to changing our gut

(continued)

bacteria, and that can, in turn, have an influence on inflammation in our bodies and on our mood. It is so important to take a look at what is in our food, water, and environment.

It wasn't until I had my own children that I started to pay close attention to the products I was applying to my skin and then the skin of my newborns. Along with phthalates, there are many other chemicals such as parabens (used as preservatives); flame retardants; and triclosan, a chemical found in products labeled *antimicrobial,* that is used in some bodywashes and other products to kill or stop the growth of germs such as bacteria and that can cause long-term harm to our children. Now I read labels and visit informative, evidence-based websites to help guide my purchases of personal care products to protect myself and my children:

- California Department of Public Health: https://safecosmetics.cdph.ca.gov/search/
- Environmental Working Group: http://www.ewg.org/skindeep/
- Campaign for Safe Cosmetics: http://www.safecosmetics.org/

Source: Written by Neha Pathak, MD, dipABLM, Co-chair, Global Sustainability Committee, American College of Lifestyle Medicine

Sugar

Sugar is a challenge for everyone because it can lead to inflammation and put us more at risk for diseases such as diabetes and heart disease. In fact, 1 recent study showed that those who consumed more sugar consumed about one-fifth of their calories from added sugars and had a 38% higher risk of dying from heart disease. Sugar and simple carbohydrates, such as white flour, white bread, and processed pastas that are easily broken down into sugars, can cause insulin levels to rise quickly, which can lead to peaks and valleys of insulin. This can affect the body and put us at risk for insulin resistance and diabetes.

Food Quiz: Which food contains the least sugar?

    a. Low-sugar cereal

    b. Marinara sauce

    c. Granola bar

    d. Salad dressing

    e. Dried fruit

Although they all contain some amount of sugar, the low-sugar cereal may actually contain the least. Dried fruit, such as a small box of raisins, can have up to 25 grams of sugar. Marinara sauce often has 6 to 12 grams of sugar added. The other options may be low in sugar, but it really depends on the nutrition and other added ingredients. If sugar, cane sugar, high fructose corn syrup, or any other type of syrup is listed as 1 of the first 3 ingredients, the product most likely contains too much sugar.

So what can a busy parent do to minimize their child's sugar intake? The following are 4 quick tips:

- Look at nutrition labels carefully; if sugar, or another type of sugar is 1 of the first 3 ingredients listed, choose a healthier alternative.
- Switch to fruits if your children crave sugar; apples, oranges, and bananas can provide sweetness with beneficial fiber and not the added sugars.
- Limit desserts and sugary snacks to a couple days a week such as the weekend; choose healthier dessert options such as low-sugar ice cream with fruit toppings or find a dessert recipe that contains healthier ingredients.
- Try to choose water instead of a sugary drink. Even juice drinks include a lot of sugar. When possible, choose a fruit over juice.

Processed Foods

Processed foods have been altered from their original form to boost flavor and extend shelf life. For example, a fresh strawberry contains nutrients such as fiber and plant chemicals such as polyphenols that fight disease. However, in contrast, a strawberry toaster pastry might contain fruit that has been combined with added ingredients such as sugar, additives, and preservatives that make the berries sweeter and prevent them from spoiling. Those extra ingredients can lead to weight gain and other problems when consumed in excess.

Food Quiz: Which of the following foods is likely the most processed (and least nutritious)?

> a. Bagged salads
>
> b. Salad dressings
>
> c. Canned black beans
>
> d. Frozen pizza
>
> e. Roasted nuts

The correct answer is frozen pizza. Companies often load them with salt, sugar, fats, and other additives to ensure that they taste good. Many foods are technically processed, but some, such as bagged salads, are only minimally processed. Assign your kids to be on "veggie duty" over the weekend and have them safely chop up lots of colored veggies to use during the week. Store them in the refrigerator to use when you are in a hurry. Have your children or teens create their own salads with whatever colorful toppings they want. It's fun and healthy! Sliced veggies can also be used as a great snack with hummus or low-fat ranch dip. Roasted nuts and canned beans are also convenient options that offer plenty of nutrition, but make sure to choose low-salt options for anything that is canned. If you have one or are able to purchase one, using a Crock-Pot or a multi-cooker is an easy way to cook black beans at home. Combine the black beans, water, a dash of salt, garlic, and tomatoes together for an hour in the cooker and create fun family meals together such as tacos, quesadillas, or black bean bowls with various toppings. In contrast, premade salad dressings are often loaded with salt, sugar, and additives such as thickeners. If you do purchase premade salad dressings, look for low-fat and low-sugar options.

With a little bit of brainstorming and planning, you and your children can choose simple whole-food alternatives that are more satisfying and offer more nutrients. Some healthier snack alternatives include sliced peppers and hummus, cheese sandwiches on whole-grain bread, tortilla chips and fresh salsa, sliced apples or pears, plain yogurt with a drizzle of honey, or air-popped popcorn with a light sprinkle of salt.

FOOD FOR THOUGHT: SAFETY FIRST

When possible, consider the following simple tips you can implement now to ensure your food is as safe as possible:

- When possible, eat more at home, and lean toward more fresh foods and fewer canned foods. Of course, there will be times when you have a hectic week and you find yourself choosing a less healthy option, and that is OK, as long as it is rarely.
- Run water for 2 to 3 minutes in the morning. This might be difficult to do every morning, even though experts believe it takes that long to clear the sediment. Even running it a shorter time has some benefit to it. When water sits in a pipe, especially overnight, there is more likelihood that heavy metals may corrode in it. Running the water can allow a flush of that so you don't drink anything you shouldn't.
- Use cold water, rather than warm water, to boil pasta or other foods. Warm water is more likely to have metals mixed into it. It's OK to wash your hands or shower in warm water, though, because you are not ingesting large amounts. *(continued)*

- Look at labels on packaging. The more ingredients you don't recognize, the more likely it may contain chemicals that are not the best to consume. If possible, avoid nonorganic fruits or veggies that may absorb high amounts of pesticides. These can include peaches, berries, and apples. If cost is a factor, balance the cost with buying other fruits, such as bananas, that are nonorganic but aren't high pesticide absorbers.

Reading and Understanding the Nutrition Label

Knowing how to decode nutrition facts labels (Figure 2.2) can help parents make nutrition-savvy decisions when stocking the pantry.

FIGURE 2.2
The Nutrition Facts Label

Nutrition Facts

8 servings per container
Serving size   2/3 cup (55g) — 1

Amount per serving
Calories   **230** — 2

	% Daily Value*
Total Fat 8g	**10%**
Saturated Fat 1g	**5%**
Trans Fat 0g	
Cholesterol 0mg	**0%**
Sodium 160mg	**7%**
Total Carbohydrate 37g	**13%**
Dietary Fiber 4g	**14%**
Total Sugars 12g	
Includes 10g Added Sugars	**20%**
Protein 3g	

— 3

Vitamin D 2mcg	10%
Calcium 260mg	20%
Iron 8mg	45%
Potassium 240mg	6%

— 4

* The % Daily Value (DV) tells you how much a nutrient in a serving of food contributes to a daily diet. 2,000 calories a day is used for general nutrition advice. — 5

Source: https://www.fda.gov/food/nutrition-education-resources-materials/new-nutrition-facts-label

1. **Serving size.** From this information, you can look at a single serving and the total number of servings in the package.
2. **Calories (per serving).** This amount refers to the number of calories per serving and will be a fraction of the total calories in the entire package. This can sometimes feel as if a food item contains fewer calories than it really does, so make sure to consider the serving size.
3. **Natural and added sugars and sodium.** These nutrients should be limited. Additionally, saturated fat and trans fat are important nutrients to limit as well.
4. **Beneficial nutrients.** This will tell you the daily value percentage of vitamins A, C, D, and E, as well as calcium, iron, magnesium, etc, included in the food.
5. **% Daily Value.** Look at all of the *% Daily Values* on the right side of the label. All the percentages indicate how much of each nutrient is in a serving when compared with the daily recommended value of 2,000 calories. For example, the recommendation is to avoid foods that have a high daily value percentage of sodium. For food items that contain sodium and saturated fat, stick to the *less than 5* rule. For nutrients, such as vitamins and minerals, look for *greater than 5%*.

Other Labels

Some simple ways to avoid the chemicals that can be in plastics such as bisphenol A (BPA) is to screen products such as baby bottles to make sure they are labeled as non-BPA. Although BPA is only 1 potentially toxic chemical found in plastic, at least it's 1 we can avoid. Additionally, you may try to transition your home to be as nonplastic as possible. This could include using glass containers instead of plastic to store food. If you do use a plastic container, do not microwave foods in it, as this can potentially cause leaching of the plastics and chemicals into your food. Similarly, don't put hot liquids such as coffee or soup into plastic containers, as hot liquids can cause leaching as well.

It is important to pay attention to labels that suggest that products are *natural* or *green*. These labels are not vetted by any regulatory agency, so the most important thing is to look on trusted websites for products that have an evidence base for safety and effectiveness. It may be very important to you to use sustainably sourced products and products with fewer human-made chemicals, and this is completely reasonable. The key, however, is to make sure that you are not buying an unsafe product because of a label that may not clearly describe the ingredients of the product. Paying attention to environmental hazards is necessary for us as parents, as well as for our children, to avoid stressing the body in any way and to set our children on a path toward a healthy future.

Power Foods: Good for the Body and the Brain

Power foods stand out because they contain large amounts of the nutrients our bodies require to maintain good health. The following are some rules of thumb that I use to select the most nutritious options for my own family:

- **Color is key.** Anything that has reds and blues in it is generally good for you. Blueberries, cherries, plums, and red grapes contain polyphenols that have anti-inflammatory actions. If it's winter, frozen berry mixes are good to toss into a smoothie as a healthy snack or dessert.
- **Root options.** Foods that are root based are good selections for optimal health. This includes carrots, turnips, radishes, sweet potatoes, ginger, and turmeric.
- **Lots and lots of greens.** I know you've heard this before, but it's worth sharing again—leafy greens such as kale, collards, and brussels sprouts contain a lot of powerful nutrients,

including folate, carotenoids, and glucosinolates, all of which may prevent diseases such as cancer. Other vitamins such as calcium and vitamin K are instrumental in bone building.

Can Foods Affect Our Mood?

We've heard about how nutrition can help build healthier bodies and better physical health, but now there is research to show that certain foods can affect our mood as well. This has to do with our gut bacteria. Some good gut bacteria produce neurochemicals such as dopamine and serotonin that can affect our emotions and can even affect the likelihood of depression. In fact, a study that looked at more than 10,000 people over 7 years found that those who ate more fruits and vegetables seemed to report greater happiness.

AROUND THE WORLD

Researchers have found that various cultures around the world have specific food traditions. Studies show that Okinawa, Japan, for example, has an especially large number of people who live to age 100 and beyond. Meals there emphasize plant foods such as orange and purple sweet potatoes, beans, and yellow and green vegetables, along with fish and green tea. A diet that is based on mostly vegetables and fish, as well as a lot of physical activity and low stress, is believed to contribute to living to a higher age. In Ikaria, Greece, another locale known for good health, the diet includes an abundance of fruits and vegetables, including greens flavored with lemon and olive oil, as well as beans such as lentils and chickpeas, and some fish. Coffee is a beverage of choice. Some cuisine in India stands out for focusing on vegetables, lentils, small quantities of yogurt, and anti-inflammatory anti-oxidant spices such as turmeric. Turmeric is used abundantly in typical Indian cooking, and yogurt or dahi is often made at home

(continued)

and served with any meal that has a lot of spice. It is also used to make lassi, a sweet yogurt drink that goes well with heavier foods such as chicken tikka masala or chana masala. My grandmother often was confused when the original dietary pyramid came out. It recommended very little fat, including very little olive oil and nuts. She didn't understand why unsaturated fats were bad when they were consumed for thousands of years in India. Today, we know that "healthy fats" are naturally occurring fats in foods such as almonds, avocados, and nuts.

Check out Table 2.1 for some useful tips I use as a mom to help offer healthy foods and meals to my children as often as possible.

TABLE 2.1
Smart Health Tips

1. The Essential 3	The Essential 3 refers to a protein, a fruit, and a vegetable. It's a success if you can eat or offer at least 1 of the essential 3s in every meal. Don't beat yourself up if you can't offer all 3 at every meal every single day.
2. How Do You Want Your Sugar?	This is a good question to ask your children at the start of every day. If they choose lemonade with lunch, that is their sugar for the day. Desserts should not be offered every day; if they would like a snack after dinner, consider whole fruit if they have a sweet craving.
3. Always Offer Water	Oftentimes, kids may think they are hungry when they are actually thirsty. Have them drink a glass of water first, and if they are still hungry, then they can choose a healthy snack.
4. Time-saver	If financially feasible, consider having your groceries shipped so you can use that time to cook and prepare 2 to 3 meals that will last you and your family well into the week. For example, you can plan for a quick-fix meal with prechopped veggies and/or meat on Monday, leftovers on Tuesday, create your own pizzas or stuffed tacos on Wednesday, and so on. Don't forget to treat yourself occasionally; who doesn't like a meal out at a restaurant once in a while?
5. Veggie Meal Prep	Precut veggies on Sunday for a quick meal or snack anytime during the week. If you make these foods easily accessible, kids will be less inclined to reach for the unhealthy options.

Fundamental 2—Quality Sleep

Parents often ask me how to protect their children and prevent them from getting sick. Although the obvious answers always include good handwashing, proper nutrition, and regular exercise, the 1 answer that people often seem to prioritize the least is adequate sleep. Sleep has a profound effect on our children and is required to help boost our immune system and fight infection.

Sleep Quiz: How many hours of sleep should a child aged 9-11 aim for?

    a. 6 hours of uninterrupted sleep

    b. 9 hours, but it's OK if it's occasionally interrupted

    c. 9-11 hours of uninterrupted sleep

The correct answer is c.

When school and social activities demand so much of our children's lives, the amount and quality of sleep they get is often sacrificed. Whether it's staying up late to finish homework, getting up early for sports training, or simply having excessive screen time or digital media use, not getting enough sleep each night can affect more than just how tired we are the following day. According to the National Sleep Foundation, only one-third of teens in the United States get enough sleep. Teens need about 9 to 10 hours of sleep, and preteens need 10 to 11. A good night's sleep can make a significant difference in our child's overall well-being by increasing energy and enhancing their focus throughout the day.

Devin

Sleep has a huge effect on emotional well-being, focus, and even physical health. When Devin came in for a well-child visit, his mom explained how Devin was experiencing low energy and lethargy while at school for several weeks. I asked lots of questions, including ones related to their daily schedule.

(continued)

Devin's mom admitted that the family schedule had been hectic: she had a new job teaching night classes, and Devin's bedtime was not consistent. At 10:00 pm, Devin was often still awake, playing video games. She agreed that Devin was probably running on too little sleep. We talked about sticking to a consistent schedule and powering down screens earlier in the evening to ensure a healthy amount of sleep every night. The next time I saw Devin and his mom, Devin shared that he was feeling more energetic and happier.

Sleep Effects on Mental Health

Mood shifts in teens are often due to hormonal changes during puberty. But these shifts are compounded by lack of sleep. In 1 study at the University of Pittsburgh, 35 children and teens were divided into 2 groups. One group was allowed to sleep only a few hours, and the other group received a full night's sleep. On a depression symptom screening test, those with limited sleep exhibited more depressive symptoms. Adequate sleep is key to help reduce the risk of mental health issues. Lack of sleep can also affect how we perceive things, positively or negatively. I admit that, even as an adult, I see things from more of a negative lens if I haven't slept well. In fact, when I am cranky, they will often ask me if I slept OK. I remember receiving an email from a colleague 1 day after a night of poor sleep and assuming that he was annoyed with me. The next day, after a full night's sleep, I read it again and was surprised to discover that there was nothing negative in the email at all. The amount of sleep we get can often alter the way we look at situations and relate to others.

Sleep Recommendations

I have found that many parents of newborns are very attentive to their infant's sleep needs but may pay less attention to sleep as their children enter elementary and middle school. This may be because life becomes more hectic with activities, kids become more independent, and it's hard to keep track of their sleep, but it is essential. Most school-aged children and teens need about 9 to 10 hours of sleep a night to function at their best. And just as too little sleep is harmful, sleeping too much can be problematic as well. Figure 2.3 outlines the specific sleep recommendations for children at each age.

FIGURE 2.3
Daily Sleep Recommendations for Infants, Children, Teens, and Adults

Age[a]	Hours per 24 Hours on a Regular Basis
4 to 12 months	12 to 16 hours (includes naps)
1 to 2 years	11 to 14 hours (includes naps)
3 to 5 years	10 to 13 hours (includes naps)
6 to 12 years	9 to 12 hours
13 to 18 years	8 to 10 hours
18 years and older	7 or more hours

[a] Recommendations for infants younger than 4 months are not included due to the wide range of normal variation in duration and patterns of sleep.

Source: Reused with permission. Table originally published in the patient education booklet *Healthy Ways to Manage Stress and Live Well* © 2021 American Academy of Pediatrics.

The following sleep tips can have a huge effect on your child's overall well-being and happiness:

Sleep Tip 1—Pretty simple: be a zealot about sleep. Yes, I just said that because sleep is key. Make sure that at least 2 or 3 days a week your kids or teens sleep the full 10 hours they need. This may mean cutting down some activities or socialization. In our home, during the school year, we've not only cut out screen time Monday through Thursday but also sleepovers during weekdays and even on the weekends. Sleepovers are now allowed on long weekends and holidays only. It took some adjusting, but my kids are more well rested. They seem happier and enjoy anticipating and planning those special occasion sleepovers. Take a look at what you can change in order for your children to receive the rest they need.

Sleep Tip 2—Reconsider a full schedule. Does your child need to be in 3 sports? Which activity is not bringing them complete happiness? Although it's healthy for kids to experience various sports and activities, and not specialize in just 1, a packed schedule can lead to stress and even a lack of enjoyment. Late afternoon sports and practices can often push homework and bedtimes later. Teens know to make time for homework and projects but may struggle to find that time when they are signed up for multiple activities or sports. Talk with your child and determine which activity, hobby, or sport makes them most happy and what can be let go. Ultimately, this can feel relieving to your child, knowing they have time for tasks that are required and can look forward to activities they enjoy without the added pressure of a busy schedule.

Sleep Tip 3—Reduce your child's use of devices. Yes, this means the tablet, their cell phone, and TV to eliminate unnecessary distractions. Devices need to be turned off 1 hour before bedtime if possible. Avoid placing a TV in their bedroom. Sometimes online homework can interfere with a screen time limitation, but encourage your child to complete it earlier in the evening whenever possible.

Fundamental 3—Water and Hydration

Have you or your child ever felt sluggish in the afternoon and reached for a kick of caffeine to give your focus a boost? What if 2 glasses of water could give you that same energy back?

Multiple studies on dehydration showed that even mild dehydration can affect focus and energy. Keeping hydrated by drinking water can help our kids perform better at school, while assisting with executive functioning.

Athletes have a strong understanding of hydration. They drink water and replenish electrolytes constantly, which affects their performance. Most people need about 6 to 8 glasses of water a day, but in reality, most do not drink this much water.

The following are some quick changes you can make with your kid to increase their hydration:

- Have your kid drink a big glass of water when they get up first thing in the morning. Most of us are dehydrated in the morning, and drinking a glass of water can help replenish what we lost overnight.
- Offer a glass of water with every meal. If your kid eats 3 meals a day, they will have at least 3 glasses of water each day.
- If your kid reaches for a sugary drink or juice instead of water, ask them to choose between the sugary drink or dessert (this can only work on dessert day, of course).
- Make sure your kid brings a water bottle to school and to any athletic activity.

THE RISK OF LEAD

One myth that many believe is that lead contamination only happens in old homes or in older cities like Flint, Michigan. Unfortunately, this is not true. An investigation soon after the crisis in 2014 showed that more than 3,800 neighborhoods across the United States had high lead levels, some with levels that were double those found in Michigan in 2014. Lead levels can be elevated because, even in new buildings and in new

(continued)

houses, the water still is coming through old service lines beneath the ground. Often in these service lines, the old pipes are eroded, which leads to the toxic heavy metal as well as other contaminants coming into our drinking water.

Unfortunately, the effects of lead on a child's body are vast, and although there is no real cure to reverse the effects, the sooner you are aware of the common places lead may be found, the better able you are to avoid exposure. Body harm from lead includes almost every system, including the vascular system, bones, and kidneys. For young children, lead can cause harm to the developing brain. It can cause behavioral issues, such as the symptoms found in attention-deficit/ hyperactivity disorder, and hearing loss and can affect IQ. Also, hearing and speech problems can affect learning, leaving kids behind academically at an early age.

The best way to prevent your child from drinking toxins is to be aware of what is in your water. The good news is that lead poisoning and toxicity are preventable. The first thing a parent can do is determine whether there is an issue of contaminated water in your area. You can also find out if there is a lead service line bringing water into your home. Although some systems might have issues, most will be OK. If you are concerned, talk to your water company about the treatment that the water gets. You can also test the water in your home and check to see if your school district uses clean water if kids are drinking out of a fountain. Other options include installing a water filter under the sink or alternatively using a water filter pitcher.

Other possible sources of lead exposure include dust from old paint. If your home was built before 1978, it could have paint that has lead underneath other layers of paint. If you decide to do a renovation, make sure that your contractor knows lead-safe practices and has been certified by the US Environmental Protection Agency. Home kits that test for lead can help, but they test only the surface, not the layers of paint beneath.

Fundamental 4—Move Your Body Through Exercise

We know that exercise helps us stay healthy, maintain a healthy weight, and helps prevent many diseases. Exercise does not always have to mean going to the gym, buying the most expensive weights and equipment, or running a marathon. Exercise is anything that moves the body and can include games, chores, and play. Children and youth (5-17 years of age) should aim to engage in about 60 minutes of daily activity. This does not have to be all at once but can be spread out throughout the day such as 6 activities of 10 minutes each. If children are not able to achieve this goal right away, they can work together with their parents to work toward it gradually.

Inflammation is the cause of many diseases, including those that can affect our memory. In 1 study, only 20 minutes of moderate exercise decreased the production of tumor necrosis factor, an inflammatory chemical in the body that can increase the risk of diabetes and even cancer. In another study, older adults who exercised regularly showed better memory function than those who did not. If this is helpful in brains that are older, imagine the response that a developing brain such as that in our children could have. Exercise works!

Exercise can also alter mood. In a recent study published in a medical journal, data showed that 15 minutes of running or 1 hour of brisk walking reduced the risk of depression. Moving the body releases endorphins, often within 5 minutes, which can literally make you or your kids feel better. Movement is an essential part of improving focus and energy. Exercise can help distract you from certain worries and stressful parts of your life. It is much harder to move forward with stressful or negative thoughts while trying to walk, run, play, or complete a yoga class. Your mind has a chance to take a break and focus on the physical activity. Once you've had a break from the cycle of anxiety, you can return to your activity with more focus and improved energy.

It's not easy to encourage preteens and teens to move outside of organized sports. The following tips are a few of my favorite strategies to incorporate fun physical activity into your family life.

Movement Tip 1—Exercise with your kids. Yes, you heard me! It doesn't work if you sit on the couch. Make it about the family, and plan a 15-minute run or a 30-minute walk. Start small and build up.

Movement Tip 2—Rename the movement! Calling it something other than *exercise* or *physical activity* will prevent you from thinking of this time as a chore, drudgery, or something to check off your to-do list for the day. Is it a playlist dance party? Is it a game of hoops, or throwing the football around? Whatever works, label it as such instead of as *exercise*, and you will raise your heart rate and move your body while also having fun!

Movement Tip 3—Working out doesn't have to be expensive. For teens, digital apps work great. If they are old enough to ride a stationary bike or run on the treadmill, set up the online class for them. Classes are widely available online for free or for a small monthly fee on digital workout apps without having to own the expensive equipment. Some classes don't even require any equipment at all. Let them decide whether they'll complete a 15-minute or 30-minute session. If they have some control over how they exercise (with a fun playlist!), they're more likely to make it happen.

Movement Tip 4—Look for ways to improve exercise. Some types of exercise can provide double the benefits. For example, yoga is a physical form of exercise that has a range of positive benefits for stress, anxiety, depression, coping, and other psychological factors. Online yoga classes are also widely available. These classes would be a good idea after dinner to provide movement and help children wind down as bedtime approaches. (But ensure that screens are shut down at least an hour before bedtime.)

Exercise acts as a form of medicine and can provide benefits to all age groups. This fundamental is not easy, especially when your schedules are jam-packed, but if you engage in exercise as a family, it will be a smoother adjustment and will help you as much as the kids. Regularly changing up your movement routine can help prevent boredom and make it more appealing and fun.

Slow Down and Recharge

It seems nearly impossible to slow down when society encourages us to think and be faster, harder, and stronger. But when we slow down, and allow ourselves to recharge, we actually are able to refuel and become more productive.

As a parent, have you had a very hectic week, and then on the weekend you had little scheduled? I certainly have. And you know what? It really helped me to have that downtime. Similarly, kids need downtime as well. It may seem silly to build in or schedule time to recharge, but it can help your children refuel and tackle future activities with a more focused, calmer mindset. Prioritize what's important to you and your family, and make sure recharging is part of that schedule.

Finding Your Way Back to the Basics

Grounding yourself and your family with these important fundamentals can help us as parents reset what our children need to make them happy, healthy, and successful. It's not easy to adjust life to do this, especially with all the pressures that are associated with society's definition of success. But practicing them as a family and doing them together when your kids are young or as preteens and teens will help them form good habits that can help them when they are older. Lifestyle changes can set the foundation for building what is most important—kids who are healthy, strong, and resilient and able to pivot in an ever-changing world.

Toolbox Takeaways for Embracing the Fundamentals

TAKEAWAY 1: **Check-in**

Have a devices spot in the kitchen or somewhere away from bedrooms. At an agreed-on time (at least an hour before bedtime), have your kids check in their devices. Even better, do it yourself, too, to set a good example. This will help everyone get uninterrupted sleep.

TAKEAWAY 2: **Nutrition**

As you throw together dinner, place an open bag of baby carrots on the counter alongside a container of hummus for hungry kids to graze. This boosts their veggie intake and minimizes the chances of them snacking on unhealthy foods.

TAKEAWAY 3: **Time Saving**

When financially possible, consider grocery delivery services. You can submit your order online, which saves time. (And many sites allow you to repeat previous orders, making the process even faster.) This promotes healthy eating because you're not tempted to buy junk food or engage in impulse purchasing.

TAKEAWAY 4: **Hydration**

Treat everyone in the family with a snazzy new water bottle. Some fun ones are available online that feature measurement lines, often with funny sayings, that encourage you to maintain drinking so you drink the required amount per day.

TAKEAWAY 5: **Exercise**

Ask your teen to search social media for short at-home workout videos you can do together at least once a week. This takes the prep out of your hands, places control in your kid's, and gives your family a new way to move and connect.

QUIZ

Is Your Family Overscheduled?

1. How many days of the week does your child have free time and can decide how to spend their time?
   - a. Most days (0 points)
   - b. A few times a week (2 points)
   - c. Once a week (3 points)
   - d. Never (5 points)

2. How many days do you manage to eat 1 meal together as a family?
   - a. Most days (0 points)
   - b. A few times (2 points)
   - c. Once (3 points)
   - d. Never (5 points)

3. How often does your child turn in school assignments on time?
   - a. Most of the time (0 points)
   - b. About half of the time (3 points)
   - c. Almost never (5 points)

4. How often is your child resistant to heading to an extracurricular activity?
    a. Never (0 points)
    b. Occasionally, but not often (1 point)
    c. About half the days of the week (3 points)
    d. Most of the time (5 points)

5. How do you as a parent feel about running your child to their next activity?
    a. I don't feel too bad about it. (0 points)
    b. It's not my favorite thing, but I can tolerate it. (3 points)
    c. I could scream or cry: #overit. (5 points)

Add up your score. Total _____

What Your Score Means

0 to 8 points: Thumbs up! You and your family are managing schedules well, which helps everyone's physical and mental health. Keep your eyes on the prize. Continue to schedule downtime and prioritize family connection.

9 to 16 points: You're trying your best to prevent your child from being overscheduled, although some days are more successful than others. Take a look at your schedule periodically to determine how you can reclaim a little time in the day. Are all activities on the schedule absolutely necessary? Can the whole family agree to put down screens and get outside?

17 to 25 points: Your family appears to be in the overscheduling danger zone. No doubt most of you are feeling squeezed, frazzled, and tired. Something's got to give. Give your schedule a serious look and make some hard choices about what can be put on hold or dropped so everyone can transition into a healthier place.

CHAPTER 3

The Loss of Unscheduled Time

There are many drivers when it comes to overscheduling. One of the main factors is our cultural expectation that kids should excel in all areas, including academics, sports, and other extracurricular activities, all while maintaining busy social lives. In the sports arena, parents often believe that it's essential for our kids not only to participate in a sport but also to train to be a star. There's the constant urge to do everything and the pressure of FOMO (*fear of missing out*) fueled by the comparisons of other people and families who post on social media. It's hard to resist the temptation to compare our children and family life to others' while scrolling through various social media platforms. And for many families, there's the pressure of looming college applications and the sense that our kids are somehow falling behind. As a parent and pediatrician, I say that it's time for a reality check.

THE PANDEMIC OF 2020

Arun was in eighth grade and was in soccer 4 times a week, including 3 practices after school and games on the weekend. He loved it, but also being on the debate club and the yearbook committee, he barely had time to eat dinner and finish his homework. Most nights he would not get to bed until 11:00 pm. It felt doable for the first 2 months of school, but when math started becoming more difficult to understand, Arun began to struggle. Soon Arun started turning in assignments late—and eventually missing them altogether. By the second semester, he felt as if he were drowning. Arun had always been an excellent student and felt too ashamed to ask his parents for help. When his activities were canceled during the COVID-19 pandemic, he finally felt that he could take a breath. It was during this time he realized he needed to cut back.

The Truth About Youth Sports

The benefits of sports are not a mystery. Sports keep kids moving with regular physical activity that benefits both body and mind. Team participation gives them a way to connect with peers. And working hard on drills and completing training runs teaches kids that practice and dedication can pay off.

At the same time, youth sports can have a flip side. As sports have grown more competitive at younger ages, a growing number of kids are experiencing injuries, often the result of overuse. The number of high school baseball players undergoing "Tommy John" surgery, which repairs the ligament that ties together the bones of the elbow, has increased rapidly in teens aged 15 to 19. The popularity of soccer is one reason that the rate of anterior cruciate ligament tears in kids' knees has increased by 2.3% per year for 2 decades. And 1 in 5 teens in contact sports have experienced at least 1 concussion. These injuries suggest that kids are being pushed too hard at young ages, leading to injuries that could affect them for life. Youth sports has grown into a $19 billion industry. Families are often expected to spend thousands of dollars each year for fees, equipment costs, and travel, limiting families with a lower income.

A growing number of children are finding team sports stressful. A 2019 survey by the Aspen Institute found that the average kid spends less than 3 years playing a sport and quits by age 11 because it's no longer fun. The Aspen Institute launched the "Don't Retire, Kid" campaign, hoping to help kids rediscover the fun of sports, in part by reintroducing unstructured free play and encouraging them to sample different sports to prevent burnout. This approach also helped them avoid overuse injuries. If your child wants to try multiple sports, I suggest that they try activities that meet in different seasons.

Sports aren't the only activities that can become overwhelming if not managed properly. Any extracurricular activity, such as band, drama, cheerleading, or the school paper, can become a source of stress if your child never gets a break and feels unrelenting pressure. The following ideas can help maintain healthy attitudes about extracurricular activities.

- **Check in periodically.** Ask your child if they are having fun. Keep the lines of communication open and encourage them to share with you if they are not enjoying the activity, it feels too stressful, or they simply do not want to continue. Converse with your kids and talk about the option to stop and walk away if that's what they prefer.

- **Be your child's parent, not their coach.** To avoid creating excessive stress or unnecessary pressure around your children's performance while in sports, allow them to initiate conversations after games. I particularly like this advice from the Aspen Institute's Project Play, which recommends that every conversation about your child's sport include the sentence, "I love to see you play." Comment and praise them on their efforts and not on whether they scored a goal or touchdown or whether they won the game or not.

- **Be realistic.** Statistics from the National Collegiate Athletic Association reveal that only 2% of high school athletes are offered athletic scholarships to college, so adjust your expectations. Given that reality, is the elite traveling team a must? Maybe it's enough for your kid to let them have fun and exercise on a recreational team with smaller fees and a limited time commitment.

The Stress of Seeking Academic Success

Academic expectations usually begin to ramp up in middle school. In some communities, the pressure to excel can be extreme, and good grades are considered an important step to be accepted into colleges. Additionally, the number of college applications has increased so much that many parents feel competitive pressure for their kids to get admitted to college. In 2001, the No Child Left Behind legislation was introduced and required schools to administer standardized tests in reading and math annually for grades 3 through 8 and once during high school. Schools reported their results for all students and for particular groups, including English learners and students in special education, racial minorities, and children from low-income families. Schools were required to hit annual achievement targets, and those that didn't faced sanctions that grew more severe each year they fell short.

Educators say this high-stakes pressure led many teachers to teach a curriculum aligned with the tests. Many schools boosted the amount of homework they gave students and eliminated classes such as music, physical education, art, and even history and social studies so they could spend more time on test topics. No Child Left Behind was eventually reworked years later, requiring fewer penalties for struggling schools, but standardized tests still remain in many schools.

Academic pressure often increases as kids enter high school. Some college-bound students take challenging Advanced Placement courses and are required to take the SAT or ACT for admission to a specific college. Interestingly, the 2020 coronavirus pandemic may have led some top universities, including Cornell and Harvard, to waive the SAT and ACT requirements for admission, at least temporarily. Other universities, such as the California state system, have pledged to eliminate the SAT and ACT as an admissions requirement over the next 4 years. Critics of the tests say they give more affluent students an advantage because their families can afford expensive test preparation programs.

Developing Realistic Expectations

I encourage parents to foster healthy attitudes about academics. We want our kids to succeed, and to have the best opportunities available, but at what cost? If you've ever sat at the kitchen table with a fourth grader crying about the book report they have to finish before bed, or the seventh grader feeling defeated by the B they received on a math test, you know the need for balance. As a parent, you can influence how your child thinks about academics and grades and help them develop realistic expectations for themselves. Is it reasonable to expect an A in every subject? Despite what kids might think, it's not true that "everyone" is succeeding in every class; also, this may not even be a reasonable goal. Grades are important, but it's more important that your child aims to do quality work. Mistakes are normal and expected; perfection is not.

It may help to chat with other parents and find families with similar struggles. One mom I know was alarmed by the amount of homework her fifth grader, Olivia, received. Olivia struggled to finish all of the assigned work on a weekly basis. It wasn't until her mother began talking to other parents that she learned she wasn't the only one concerned about the homework load and the fact that it involved several hours on a screen. Other parents were equally concerned and worked with teachers to come up with shorter, nonscreen alternatives for homework.

Managing Academic Expectations

If you are someone who has always been driven and want your kids to be academic stars, it may be wise to manage your expectations as a parent. This can be a little difficult, but I encourage parents to be honest with themselves about their child's strengths and to fight the urge to compare their kids with those of friends or siblings. This kind of thinking can push kids into classes or activities that are beyond their abilities and increase their anxiety and stress levels.

Parents may want to avoid micromanaging their kid's homework and, instead, help them develop the skills to complete projects on their own, which will pay off in the long run, as they progress through their academic career. For example, you might ask your child how long they estimate it will take to write the essay or complete their math homework, and then talk them through the process of deciding the best time to start working. Over time, your kids can learn to plan their work in this way without your help.

HOMEWORK STRUGGLES

If your child or teen struggles with homework or fights with you about completing it, reach out to their teacher or school counselor. Explain that your kid is having difficulty and ask if the teacher or counselor can suggest strategies to help. Ensuring a good and communicative relationship with your child's teacher can be very beneficial when ensuring your child's academic needs are addressed. This can also take the pressure off you, ease fights at home, and help preserve your relationship with your kid. The state of your relationship could make all the difference in your kid's stress level.

In middle school and high school, try to work with your kids and guide them through organization and work habits. For example, if your kid performs poorly on a test, view it as a learning opportunity for them. Encourage them to understand why they got that grade and what it was that they didn't understand. They may figure out that it would be helpful to approach the teacher before or after school for extra help. This will give them an opportunity to self-advocate, which is key in life. If the reason was that they made careless mistakes, then help them recognize how to avoid those mistakes in the future and strategize ways to stay focused. Always frame feedback in positive ways, and praise your kids for the efforts they've put in rather than the grade.

When it comes to standardized testing, it's important to help your child without creating more pressure. Many families may not have the means to afford private tutors, but it doesn't mean that their kid can't succeed. For the tests, try beginning the studying process early. There are many preparation books available and online programs, too. Use these with your kids, and if your child has test-taking anxiety, start preparing even earlier. Practice with trial tests and make sure your child is comfortable with timing. Parental calmness around the tests can make a real difference to kids' stress levels and can continue to provide perspective. "Do your best, forget the rest," is a good mantra. The reality that college is only 1 step in life's journey can help everyone have clarity and add some grounding as you and your family navigate a stressful time.

Too Little Unscheduled Time

With increased time focused on standardized test topics and evenings and weekends rushing from homework to sports to music lessons to theater practice, little to no unstructured downtime is available for play and creativity. Not only does playfulness serve as an important buffer against stress but it can also help children develop the social and cognitive skills and imagination required in a world that values innovative thinkers.

Results from a University of Colorado study showed that children with more unstructured time had better executive functioning, meaning that they were better able to solve problems and make decisions. One mother once shared with me that she scheduled an after-school playdate for her 7-year-old son in the midst of a busy week. When she picked him up at school and announced that they were headed over to play with his friend, he burst into tears, pointing out that he'd already had piano and swim lessons and religious education that week, which hadn't left any time to play in his room. It was an eye-opening moment for his mother, who said she finally understood how much he needed that unstructured time and viewed it as an important lesson about safeguarding her son's downtime.

The Importance of Time to Replenish

As parents, we are cognizant of the benefits of time to ourselves: When we rest, we not only feel better but also are more likely to have the energy to think outside the box and be creative. Most of us can think of a time when we've "slept" on a problem and the next morning woke up with a clear mind and possible solutions. Giving our minds some space can allow us to make connections and dream up ideas that don't occur to us in the hubbub of a busy day, and the same can be true for our children.

In a 2019 essay in the *New York Times,* entitled, "Let Children Get Bored Again," writer Pamela Paul points to a survey indicating that parents often feel guilty when kids say, "I'm bored," leading parents to believe this means they haven't done enough to provide enriching activities. "Every spare moment is to be optimized, maximized, driven toward a goal," Paul wrote.

But in reality, being bored may be a catalyst for creative thinking. In the essay, she noted that composer and actor Lin-Manuel Miranda of *Hamilton* fame credits long, unsupervised afternoons in his childhood with sparking inspiration. Another study revealed that people who completed mindless tasks were especially creative during a later task. This is an interesting idea for us as parents: allowing kids the opportunity to do mundane (and helpful!) chores such as mowing the lawn or unloading the dishwasher might actually stimulate creative ideas. It's yet another way that helping around the house is beneficial to kids.

Making Time to Help Others

Many schools are introducing social and emotional learning into their curriculum. There are many benefits with these programs for kids, families, and communities, such as helping kids develop empathy and concern for others. Research shows that children who show empathy are less likely to bully, more likely to have academic and career success, and more likely to develop positive relationships. And helping others through good deeds such as volunteering at a food pantry or animal shelter provides myriad health benefits, including a reduced risk of depression. People who volunteer may experience "the helper's high," or positive feelings as a result of serving others. Especially during stressful periods, it can be healing to direct our attention outward to help others.

It may seem strange, in a chapter about overscheduling, to suggest that families add additional activities such as volunteering to their weekly routine. But I feel strongly that this is time well spent. Making a family commitment to use some of your free time, when available, to help others can bring more positivity, gratitude, and compassion into your life.

It's important to teach children that even the smallest of acts can really mean a lot. They might spend a few hours on a Saturday morning at the local food pantry or humane society or reach out to a great-aunt who lives alone. Acts of kindness can be as simple as washing a neighbor's car or shoveling their driveway after a snowstorm or sharing part of a batch of cookies with a friend. Tweens and teens often have surprisingly good ideas of ways to give back to others. A family friend of mine gifted her beloved doll and accessories to a younger girl in the neighborhood and spent an hour with her showing her the doll's outfits.

The Positives of Saying No: Listening and Learning

Most adults can think of times when they said yes to something they wished they'd declined. They know the feeling that settles in when committing to evening plans after an already busy day, taking on more responsibilities outside of work, or even canceling your own personal plans for last-minute changes or friend requests. Saying no can be very hard! If you find yourself struggling to say no, reflect on why; you might think that saying yes often ensures that others will like you, or you worry that you'll be criticized for not pulling your weight. Becoming comfortable with saying no is 1 of the most powerful tools available to free up your time and energy. Talk with your children about the importance of saying no when it's necessary, and discuss the ways that doing so provides the flexibility to say yes to the things that matter most to you and to them.

My son plays tennis, and sometimes I find myself, as a parent, pushing him to attend as often as possible. After he missed several practices because of a mild cold, I immediately pulled out the tennis tournament list and asked him if he wanted to play the following week. I was disappointed when he said no, and I asked him why. I was actually pleased with his very thoughtful answer: He said he hadn't practiced for a week and didn't want to show up unprepared. He wanted to spend the time practicing, as well as catching up on a big school project. In my rush to revert back to our busy schedule, I had slipped into my go-getter mom mode again. I was glad that my son had stopped me in my tracks. Listening to our kids is so important, and giving them a chance to weigh in really matters for their mental and physical well-being.

The Art of Making Choices

There's the saying, "The most precious resource we have is time." In our overscheduled lives, it's important to understand how making wise choices about how to spend our scheduled and unscheduled time can help kids minimize stress, increase their energy, and boost their mood.

Be brave. Be brave about saying no when it's too much. Be on guard against new activities that will overload your kid (and you). And think about how you might be able to trim back existing commitments. Maybe that dance practice won't fit in today's schedule.

Create a family calendar. Establish a shared calendar that provides the entire family a way to see what's scheduled each week. You might already have a virtual calendar accessible by smartphone, but consider a large physical calendar in a communal space such as the kitchen that is easier for younger kids to see and understand. Include everything from soccer games and work trips to family pizza night and volunteer gigs. The point of the calendar is not to attempt to make everything run with military precision but to keep parents and kids on the same page, which can reduce stress by allowing each family member to see what days are scheduled and what days they have time to relax. This can also help children figure out the best ways to spend their time and voice their concerns if something feels too much. Discuss expectations such as how many social events per week is acceptable or what time homework should be completed by. As kids enter middle school, have them add their events to the calendar. Make sure they consider driving time in order to arrive at an event on time and preparation and cleanup time around meals.

Make thoughtful discussions about time part of your ongoing family conversation. When kids express interest in a new team or club or want to attend an event such as a ski trip, help them to think through the time it will involve and review the calendar together to see if adding the event would add stress. What other activities might they need to miss or shift if they opt for this new activity or event? Ask your kids what they consider their top priorities.

Prioritize family time. Make daily downtime and family time a priority when planning your week. Be religious about scheduling these items before you commit to other obligations. When my kids were preteens, we often scheduled 2 to 3 hours on Sunday morning or afternoon to spend time together, with our phones and computers shut down. It's a bit harder now that they are teens and have more homework, but I still insist on finding some quality family time with minimal device use on the weekends. According to the Clay Center for Young Healthy Minds at Massachusetts General Hospital, "For children, spending time with tough coaches is far less enriching than spending time with a mom or dad who enjoys their company. This bolsters their self-esteem more effectively than anything else."

Limit activities. Consider enacting a rule that each child can participate in only 1 major and 1 minor activity per season. In my family, we've found that more than that makes us too busy and doesn't allow enough time for academic work, rest, and family time.

Train your family to pause. Encourage everyone to form the habit of checking in with each other before agreeing to an event or activity. This is a mindful approach to scheduling and allows you to weigh and discuss obligations before agreeing to them.

Despite the many struggles the global pandemic created, for some families, it gave them a chance to reexamine how they spent their days. How did it feel to suddenly stop the race to school each morning and the car-pool duties in the afternoon? Or for some adults to halt the commute to work and business trips? What was it like to spend Saturdays without soccer and hockey and cross-country? Some families shared with me that it provided an opportunity to reconsider their schedules and even reorient their priorities. My own family and I have tried to learn the lessons from those quiet, less social days. My hope is that families can continue to be more mindful of how they spend their time, creating more downtime for thinking, napping, or spending time together.

COPING WITH THE PANDEMIC REALITY

The pandemic placed many challenges and stresses on working parents, who were forced to juggle careers with remote schooling and closed child-care centers. Some children struggled to learn under new conditions, and many missed the vital face-to-face time with their teachers and peers. Parents struggled to be as upbeat as possible to set the tone for the family as we faced new challenges. Many learned that it involved setting routines, such as keeping bedtimes and wake-up times consistent and finding multiple new ways for kids to play, learn, and interact with other people. I loved hearing about the grandchildren who set up a virtual call with their grandmother once a week for a baking lesson and the eighth graders who had a standing date on Saturday night for role-playing games. I loved the idea of 2 middle school friends who set up a dog-walking business. Walking dogs 6 feet apart while wearing masks may not have felt like old times, but it gave them a chance to see each other, engage in exercise, and earn some extra pocket money.

Toolbox Takeaways for Overscheduling

TAKEAWAY 1: **Productivity**

Schedule according to your child's most productive times (and your own). Our energy levels ebb and flow, and it can help to schedule more intense activities for the times when we're fresh. For example, if your middle schooler isn't a night owl, it's counterproductive to ask them to do math homework right before bed. Waking up 30 minutes earlier in the morning to complete it may make the process more efficient.

TAKEAWAY 2: **Breaks**

Consider scheduling hour-long, screen-free, do-nothing breaks for your kids whenever possible. That may sound like a lot of downtime, but productivity experts say that carving out that quiet time to draw or reset or read daily improves sleep and leads to more productivity and creativity in the long run. A single chunk of free time once a week is not enough to rejuvenate most busy kids.

TAKEAWAY 3: **Priorities**

When your kids are invited to a social event such as a birthday party or school dance, consider it as an activity. Limit activities to no more than 2 a day on the weekend and try to reserve 6 to 8 hours for a period of no activities. Perhaps it is a Saturday afternoon after the morning soccer game or Sundays that are reserved for downtime. Talk to your kids about why this is important; you might be surprised at how they may make this a priority, too!

TAKEAWAY 4: **Discussion**

If your child is reluctant to participate in an activity, sit them down and listen to their point of view in a calm manner. Sometimes kids will understand their circumstances even better than you do. Their reasoning may be because they are too tired to do their homework, or they are overwhelmed, similar to the way adults can feel. Listening and discussing as a team is key in making smart and healthy decisions while teaching them to be introspective.

TAKEAWAY 5: **Recovery**

Adults and children alike need to prioritize our health when our bodies tell us we need time to recover. Keep your child out of a practice or school if they are sick and let them rest. It will keep them healthy and less stressed and convey to them the importance of self-care.

QUIZ

Is Your Child's Digital Media Use Excessive?

1. When you ask your child or teen to put away their phone or shut off a screen, how hard is it for them to do?
   a. It's not hard. They generally comply. (0 points)
   b. It usually takes multiple requests for my child to power down, but they will eventually do so. (1 point)
   c. I usually need to negotiate many times and sometimes even threaten a time out. (3 points)
   d. This is one of the hardest things I ask my child to do. They resist and have been known to throw tantrums. This creates big drama in our house. (5 points)

2. Describe your child's relationship with digital devices.
   a. They don't have access to them. (0 points)
   b. They can take them or leave them. (1 point)

    c. Some days they are inseparable from
      screens, but they usually can be talked into
      switching to nonscreen activities. (3 points)
    d. Screen media are all my child seems to think
      and talk about. (5 points)

3. How often does your child's screen use interfere with
family activities? (For example, your child refuses to
come to the table for dinner or won't participate in a
family event because they are gaming.)
    a. Never (0 points)
    b. Sometimes (2 points)
    c. Often (4 points)
    d. Daily (5 points)

4. Has your child ever snuck screen use?
    a. It has not happened that I know of. (0
      points)
    b. Yes, it's happened once or twice. (1 point)
    c. Yes, this happens occasionally. (3 points)
    d. Yes, this happens regularly. (5 points)

5. Does your child ever stay awake at night to text with
friends, play video games, or view online content?
    a. No. My child's devices are located outside
      the bedroom at night, and they don't inter-
      fere with sleep. (0 points)
    b. Yes. I've found my child awake and on
      screens at least 1 time after their usual bed-
      time. (2 points)
    c. Yes. My child occasionally uses devices after
      we've said goodnight. (4 points)

      d. Definitely. Despite us having arguments
      about screens at night, my kids will
      eventually go back to sneaking their
      devices into their rooms after I go to sleep.
      (5 points)

Add up your score. Total _____

What Your Score Means

0 to 7 points: You and your child or teen are doing a good job of establishing boundaries with screen time. Nice work! Continue to talk regularly about healthy screen use, and encourage your kids to step away from screens and find in-person ways to connect with family and friends whenever possible.

8 to 18 points: Your child's screen habits can be problematic at times. It's important for you and your child to talk regularly about screen use (and how screens are designed to draw us in). Try to discourage absorption by all family members in digital devices to prevent screens from monopolizing all of your family's free time. Agreements about screen use can help.

19 to 25 points: Your child is very immersed in screens, as many kids are, and their digital media use may pose a higher risk or be problematic. It's important to have respectful conversations about screen use with your child and to discuss (and model) what the healthy use of digital devices looks like. Consider a family agreement about screen use with firm rules, such as no devices at mealtimes or bedtime. Make an effort to encourage more face-to-face time for your child with peers and family members.

CHAPTER 4

The Rise of Digital Media and the Battle for Screen-free Time

t's no surprise: Digital media is everywhere. And I know from my own family and from my work that screens and digital media are an ever-expanding part of our lives. Digital and social media have many benefits, but unfortunately they can also introduce significant risks. Many parents try to limit their children's screen time but often end up losing the battle when they become busy or under duress such as the recent pandemic. It is not always easy to moderate digital media use by kids (and adults!), and even pediatricians who are parents like me sometimes struggle. But I do believe in encouraging parents and kids to be more deliberate and mindful about their screen use and to ensure that screens don't steal time from other important and healthy activities, including homework, exercise, face-to-face social interactions, and quality rest.

Lately, I've been hearing more and more stories like Danny's—he is 14 years old and has embraced video games and gaming for many years. When he started gaming at age 9, his mom Alicia allowed him to play on Fridays and Saturdays only. But as Danny grew a social network at school and with other players on the video games, he begged for more time online. Alicia gave in because Danny's grades were good. But the slope was slippery. Eventually, Danny was online before he went to school and as soon as he got home. Alicia found herself frustrated and exhausted, constantly telling him to stop. With the demands of ninth grade, Danny's academic performance started to slip. Alicia and Danny both needed some help.

If Danny's story sounds familiar to you, and you too are constantly bumping heads with your children about screen use, it may be time to press pause on your family's current media habits. In this case, Alicia invited Danny to discuss the downsides of screen overuse and to work together on a new agreement to balance gaming and other necessary and healthy activities, including homework. Danny's involvement helped set healthy rules and encouraged his buy-in and compliance.

Unfortunately, overuse of digital media is not uncommon. Gaming, for example, has become a central activity in many teens' lives. Many kids may be interested in gaming on an even deeper level, such as becoming e-athletes. But similar to other things, if it starts affecting grades or physical or mental health, it can lead to a downward spiral. And this is certainly worth looking at together with your kids. Social media, which brings together youth and peers, is now a preferred form of communication. With newer social media platforms increasingly become more available, it has become a fact of life and part of our cultural paradigm. Another attraction of digital devices is *information hoarding*—the habit of reading news, watching videos, and consuming media obsessively. Even if kids don't actively seek out new information, features on their smartphones often push such information their way, turning every new story into a can't-miss event and tempting them to click on apps, platforms, and advertising. Overuse of digital media can lead to increased stress and anxiety in children, teens, and adults. Parents who mentor their children in healthy use of digital media can play an important role in limiting the inundation of news and discussing worrisome current events in a supportive and age-appropriate manner.

AN INCREASE IN SCREEN USE

The pandemic of 2020 shifted media use, making digital devices an even bigger part of our lives. Before the pandemic, a survey by the nonprofit Common Sense Media reported that kids 8 to 18 years old spent about 7.5 hours per day on screen-based media. But after the pandemic began in the United States in spring 2020, many schools closed and had to shift learning to online. Parents often struggled to juggle working from home via virtual meeting platforms while caring for and teaching kids. In August 2020, on NPR's "Here & Now" (https://www.wbur.org/hereandnow/2020/08/19/children-screen-time-pandemic), Michael Robb, PhD, senior director of research at Common Sense Media, said it was not yet clear how much time kids were spending on screens in this new environment. "Our best guess is that it's probably a lot more," Robb said, "because we're so much more reliant on technology than we were prepandemic."

The Appeal of Cell Phones and Social Media

Let's be honest, there are some benefits to cell phones. We as parents feel safer when we can reach our kids at any time. Kids use phones to make social connections, access a world of information right at their fingertips, and research any topic at the tap of a finger. Additionally, kids can use video chatting platforms to keep in touch with faraway relatives and friends, maintaining a level of long-distance connections that was difficult even a decade ago. But a consequence of being plugged in is that kids can be so much more aware of current news and critical topics such climate change, health, and social issues than we were growing up.

When I talk with parents about technology and social media use among kids, most say that they feel pressured to get their child a smartphone "because everyone else has one," and they don't want their child to have social difficulty because they don't have a phone. Common Sense Media surveys in 2019 revealed that more than half of US kids have a smartphone by age 11, with 1 in 5 kids receiving one by age 8. Once kids have a phone, they typically start to text, and many join social media.

The Social Media Obsession

Unfortunately, too much of a good thing is not always good. A 2015 CNN special called "#Being 13: Inside the Secret World of Teens" (https://edition.cnn.com/specials/us/being13) revealed that kids check social media more than 100 times a day, in part, child development experts say, because teens are wired to seek out peer connections. For many kids, texting and social media are a primary mode of communication with their peers. Likes and comments on social media posts provide tantalizing information about where teens stand in the valued social hierarchy.

But what are the downsides of this technology? Why do children, teens, and even we as parents, spend so much time on our devices? How do these devices affect family time and bonding? Could our time on screens promote negative physical and mental health effects, such as depression, insomnia, or even attention-deficit/hyperactivity disorder (ADHD)? Is it possible that we and our kids are becoming addicted to our devices?

This Is Your Brain on Digital Media

Addiction to digital media and its negative effects are gaining more attention from researchers and clinicians working with children and teens. Tech insiders such as Sandy

Parakilas, former platform operations manager at Facebook, describe teams of engineers who have been devoted to making social media ever more attractive and irresistible, enticing users to spend as much time as possible scrolling and clicking. Our neurobiology reinforces these habits. Research has shown that when you check your email, social media accounts, or texts, your brain releases the neurotransmitter dopamine, giving you a happy boost. After we post on social media, most of us want to check to see how others have responded. Who liked it? Who commented? Did they share it? Before you know it, you've spent an hour on the app. With each like or share comes another dopamine hit, reinforcing the habit. Imagine the effect on children, whose brains and executive function are still developing, making them more likely to be drawn in.

Our interactions online can also undermine our mental health, in part because it's so hard to resist the urge to compare ourselves to others. It can seem as if everyone online is living a better, more exciting life than yours. Even adults are susceptible to these emotions when looking at other people's beautiful vacations and incredible feasts. Kids on social media experience these images at a more vulnerable age when they may not have the ability or resources to manage their emotions.

It's also important to consider the potential effect of digital media on attention. A recent study of more than 18,000 children and teens aged 4 to 17 found that 1 in 10 have received a diagnosis of ADHD, a rise of almost 80% from data 2 decades ago. Greater awareness about and diagnosis of ADHD no doubt play a role in this observed increase, but at least 1 recent study has found links between digital media use and attention problems. The study followed 2,587 kids in 10th grade in Los Angeles for 2 years. None of the students demonstrated symptoms of ADHD at the beginning of the study, but by the end, those who used their smartphones most often were more likely to show ADHD symptoms.

Parents are not excluded from these effects either. Some have confessed to me that they, too, feel addicted to social media, which ends up taking them away from more positive interactions with their kids and other family members.

Screens Affect Communication

We've all seen this situation in restaurants, in waiting rooms, in cars, and even when kids are just hanging out: All eyes are on devices. Kids seem to be talking to each other less and are much more focused on texting, social media, and gaming. And the "tablet baby" is everywhere. A family arrives at a restaurant, the baby is seated in a high chair or toddler seat, and out comes the tablet. It's not hard to imagine that this can affect communication skills, given that communication involves reading facial expressions, voice intonations, and body language. Experts in the field underscore that much of communication is drawn from these 3 areas, but screen use does not provide an equivalent experience. Delays in vocabulary and language development have been reported that correlate with digital media use.

In 1 preliminary study of almost 900 infants and toddlers aged 6 months to 2 years, researchers found that every 30 minutes of handheld device time led to a decrease in expressive language (ie, the ability to speak words).

What about older kids, including tweens and teens? We often witness the same thing in restaurants with them using smartphones. Smartphone isolation is occurring in car pools and even at the soccer game on the sidelines, with parents watching their older child's team play while the younger sibling is looking at their phone.

A study done by the University of California, Los Angeles, examined this more closely. Two groups of sixth graders were given a test in which they were asked to look at pictures of faces and identify the emotions there, and then 1 group was sent to a device-free camp for 5 days. Both sets of kids were then asked to look at the pictures of faces again. Those who had had the screen-free time were better able to identify the emotions in the pictures than were those in the screens-as-usual group. Researchers attributed this to the break from screens and increased social interaction from camp. The study findings, suggesting that screens might blunt our ability to read cues about how other people are feeling, are worrisome. Reading those cues is an important part of kids responding well in a host of family, school, and other social situations.

In 1 study, researchers watched 55 families in fast-food restaurants and found that "a large proportion" of parents were "highly absorbed" in their devices and not connecting with their kids. We as parents need to consider how screens influence our interactions, too. Work demands, logistical concerns (who is driving the car pool next week?), and the desire to stay connected with friends mean that we're often immersed in our devices—and losing opportunities to engage with our kids.

Communication as a Tool to Help Combat Screens

There are always going to be aspects of our children's lives that will distract and divert their attention in unhealthy ways. Whether it's TV shows, movies, drugs, or alcohol, helping our children make healthy choices may feel like a constant battle. Every few years, it feels like a new technology or digital platform is created. That's why keeping communication channels open about digital media use is helpful; you and your children can learn about and address the risks and benefits of online activity together. The following tips encourage the use of open communication with your child as they engage with online followers:

- **Effects.** Talk to your children often about the effects that digital technology may have on their physical, mental, and emotional health. Do not condemn the use of digital media completely; we all know that screens are here to stay, and often kids' and teens' social circles rely on texting or other platforms. Instead, explain the risk of media overuse and how it takes away time from other necessary healthy activities. Work with your kids to develop and set ground rules for media use, and help your children comply with them.

- **Relating.** You know the saying: If you can't beat 'em, join 'em. Join 1 or 2 of the social media platforms they are using, and learn about the app. Of course, as a role model, try to avoid giving in to excessive digital media use yourself. However, spending some time seeing what their favorite apps are all about may make your discussions with your children more credible from their perspective. Ask your kids questions about which apps they like; how they are used; what they like and don't like about them; and what they feel uncomfortable about, such as oversharing, intrusiveness, or ads. These questions can open discussions so that you have insight into what's current, what's viral, what's popular, and what issues are being discussed. This kind of discussion allows parents to learn about their kids' media use so they can provide supportive guidance on healthy digital citizenship and safety online.

- **Endgame.** Ask them about what their thoughts and goals are about gaining followers and receiving likes. Do they enjoy being connected? Do they hope to be more popular among their peers and classmates? Is it because their friends have more followers? Is it because social media stars are famous or rich? When I recently had this discussion with my own kids, we identified their online hopes and wins, as well as their disappointments and possible risks. For example, they realized that they would have to invest hours and hours of time posting every day to be able to gain a following large enough for a small financial return. Asking the question, "Why are influencers and others online trying to grab your attention?" helped them think about the reasons why advertisers use advanced and hidden techniques to encourage purchases and spending. Finally, inviting them to share about how they feel while online, especially after extended media use, can help them realize that they may be experiencing more negatives than positives. Presenting and discussing the reality of digital literacy, advertising, and online use can help your children understand the risks and not just the rewards of digital media, as well as choose healthier options that comply with your family media use rules.

Digital Devices Can Make Teens Unhappy

It is clear that digital media take time away from meaningful in-person social interactions with family and friends, including activities such as family meals, tossing a ball around outdoors, or taking an after-dinner walk together. Such activities encourage face-to-face communications, closer connections with family and friends, and healthy nutrition and physical exercise. The digital world can be a harsh place, in which children and teens may see and compare themselves to idealized models, making them feel inadequate or depressed. Cyberstalking and cyberbullying can place users in danger, highlighting online connections that may be superficial and result in a greater sense of loneliness than off-line human contact does. Digital media can also be a source of frightening, unhealthy misinformation and can influence children and teens to adopt and embrace behaviors that can risk their health and lives, such as sexting, anorexia, bulimia, drug use, etc.

For that reason, I have been concerned about the recent role of media in glamorizing suicide, which is the second leading cause of death among people aged 15 to 24. In a phenomenon sometimes called *suicide contagion,* teens absorb ideas from news reports and programs. Research suggests that such exposure can increase the risk of suicide and suicidal behaviors in vulnerable media users. Therefore, in addition to providing guidance about the negative effects of digital media, I encourage you to talk with your child about suicide, what it is, and what they understand and think about it. You may feel uneasy about bringing up this subject, but it's important to have this conversation. You might use a recent suicide in your community or in TV shows or movies to launch the discussion and mention that, as some psychologists say, "depression lies" and causes people in its grip not to make the best decisions. In other words, depression can often influence the way we think. Similar to looking through a faulty physical lens with areas that are completely blocked out or blurred, looking from the viewpoint of depression can distort our perspectives and mental and emotional states.

Point out that suicide is a permanent solution to a temporary problem and that the person who died may have felt helpless or hopeless and probably didn't know that there were a lot of places to get help. Let them know that they can come to you anytime for loving help. Listen carefully to what your child is sharing so that you can provide support, assistance, and resources, if needed. If you are concerned that your child has been thinking about suicide—or planning it—call your doctor or mental health professional immediately. Chapter 8, which provides guidance for if your child is in crisis, has more information about suicide.

THE GROWING RATE OF MENTAL AND EMOTIONAL HEALTH ISSUES

Surveys reveal that many kids and teens have poor mental health. Anxiety; depression; and, disturbingly, even suicide are growing more prevalent. Between 2007 and 2014, the suicide rate doubled for kids aged 10 to 14; in girls aged 10 to 13, suicide more than tripled between 1999 and 2014. Some research suggests that digital media play a role in these heartbreaking shifts. Unfortunately, school closures and other changes during the pandemic impacted kids' mental health. According to the US Centers for Disease Control and Prevention, the emergency department visit rate for suspected suicide attempts in spring 2020 was 1.6-times higher among adults aged 18 to 25 years compared with the same time frame in 2019. Mental health–related emergency department visits during the pandemic exploded as well.

One 2018 study looked at data from more than a million teens in eighth, 10th, and 12th grade and found that, on average, those who spent more time in front of screens were less happy than those who invested more time in nonscreen activities such as sports, reading, and in-person social interactions.

Digital devices may exacerbate a child's existing vulnerabilities and mental health concerns. If your child has a tendency to be anxious, for example, the barrage of tragic headlines or a lot of intense and upsetting interactions on social media could make their anxiety flare. If your child gets overstimulated by extended screen time, then 3 hours of video games isn't the best choice. I urge parents to talk with their children to understand their experience of screen time. Ask them questions such as these: What do you enjoy about screen time? When is it hard to walk away? What is interesting or fun for you? What isn't? What bothers or upsets you? Are there ever times that spending time on a device makes you feel worse? Experts studying and providing guidance on screen use recommend that parents walk alongside their kids as they identify, address, and navigate digital media use issues, and they encourage parents to, instead of simply being media *monitors*, become media *mentors*.

The Effects of Social Media on Self-Esteem

It's important to understand the ways digital devices are shaping how teens interact with peers and feel about themselves.

Complicating how they heal. Consider a 15-year-old, in the era before social media, who breaks up with their boyfriend or girlfriend. This breakup leaves them feeling sad, but over the next month or so, the wound heals as they have little contact with their ex, and their friends and family provide support. Add social media to this picture, and the scenario can look drastically different. The ex may post negative comments about the breakup or relationship or flaunt pictures of a new significant other, dragging out the healing process. An angry ex can post online sexted photos meant to be private to humiliate their ex—photos that may stay on the internet forever. The heartbroken teen can't escape these ongoing and new wounds in the social media universe where things can be liked, shared, or commented on 24/7.

Feeling left out or lonely. Social media also create situations in which kids know when they are being left out because they see photos of what other kids are doing together. This creates fear of missing out, or FOMO, that can drive a child to check social media constantly and, ironically, contribute to loneliness. Take my friend's daughter, Melanie. She introduced her good friend to another girl, and those

2 quickly became close. When 1 of them had a birthday, Melanie's friend was invited but Melanie was not. Instead, she saw photos of the party on social media, as did other kids in the class. Photos were liked and shared, and what could have been a short, painful incident turned into a prolonged episode. As adults, most of us remember at least 1 childhood experience when we were left out, but we had the time and space to be able to move on from it. Now every log-in can reopen wounds, prevent children from healing from experiences such as this 1, and contribute to anxiety or depression.

Creating friend challenges. Another young teen I know, Beth, was having trouble with a friend who started to exclude her. When Beth would sit at the lunch table, this girl would leave for another table and convince her friends to do the same. These events were causing Beth a lot of pain. One day, Beth and her mother were scrolling through Instagram together when her mother noticed that Beth had been liking and sharing all of the girl's posts. It didn't make sense to her mother; why would Beth compliment this girl on social media? Beth explained that the girl was tracking who liked and shared her posts. She would notice if Beth didn't do so and would treat her even worse. Beth's mom was able to use this opportunity to discuss handling bullying online and off and to provide her daughter with emotional support and guidance to address middle school rejection.

Leading to unhealthy comparisons. Do you have an Instagram, TikTok, or Facebook account? If so, have you noticed how happy everyone seems to be? Travelers to exotic places, couples dressed in the latest fashions who seem to be so in love with each other, with their mansion-sized, professionally deco-rated houses. These displays can make even us adults feel deficient and deflated, believing that everyone is living a better life than ours. Unfortunately, kids and teens are even more vulnerable to believing that everyone on social media has more stuff, more friends, and a more exciting life. As a digital mentor, you can help your children learn that a lot of social media content is an illusion; those video clips are typically staged and don't reflect reality. Ask your children how many pictures they take before choosing 1 to post. Do they opt for photos taken when they look their best? Or post about the positives in their lives? So does everyone else. The conversation can also be an occasion to discuss family values and highlight the practice of gratitude for the positive experiences of your family.

Liking and followers dictate mood. Recently, I've been hearing my own kids chat about how many followers they have. My son was focusing on trying to figure out what helped him get more followers and how to get his posts to go viral. When he picked up more followers, he was quite happy, but when he looked a few days later and saw that that his most recent posts didn't receive many likes, he was very deflated. Sadly, many children and teens feel the same way. There is an addictive quality of being rewarded with likes that can affect our state of mind. A lack of likes can make media users feel unliked. As parents, we need to be aware of the multiple objectives of the social media industry and share that understanding with our children. Digital literacy helps families identify and understand the wizards "behind the curtain" of media whose purpose is to obtain and analyze private data, target advertising to a susceptible audience, and make a profit from information. Such knowledge can help kids interpret media more realistically.

My daughter and I had a conversation about the behavioral side of technology. After talking about it, she decided it would be smart and healthy for her to go on a media fast—in other words, to take a break from social media. She now understands how digital media can affect her emotions and self-esteem and is taking an active approach to managing her use. Her twin brother has also considered a similar strategy.

There are several ways I encourage parents to help their kids understand digital and social media and minimize the manipulation of their mental and emotional health when online:

- Start early discussions around the issues regarding social media and delay your kids' signing up for social media accounts. If they can start later (such as eighth grade), it will allow them to be more mature. A more mature brain can process more complex issues and begin to make better decisions.

- Once they do join social media, talk to them about the risks of its use in advance and ask them to come to you if they have any concerns or worries or are feeling uncomfortable or upset. You can discuss physical effects of media use, such as weight gain and sleep disturbances, as well as mental health effects such as depression.

- Turn off app notifications and develop a family media plan to provide screen time boundaries. It's critical that online activity not replace healthier needs such as exercise, independent play, homework, and face-to-face communication. The American Academy of Pediatrics (AAP) offers a family media plan template (see Resetting Our Relationship With Devices later in this chapter) that you and your family can use to prioritize healthy and necessary activities before turning to screen use for entertainment.

- Try to encourage social media breaks. Even 3 to 4 hours can provide a much-needed reset, but planning a day of

off-line, unplugged activities with family and friends can
be very refreshing.

- Let your children know that inappropriate pictures on
social media or comments can live there forever and
could have negative social and legal consequences.
Check in with them frequently about their posts and
instruct them never to share inappropriate pictures or
comments, even if they are posted by others. Encourage
them to come to you if they ever have any questions or
concerns or if they ever feel victimized.

- Discuss the risks of cyberstalking and the loss of privacy.
Encourage them never to share personal information,
including phone numbers or addresses, online. Let them
know to come to you if they are ever bullied online or
see someone else being bullied.

This Is Your Body on Digital Media

As a pediatrician, I think it's important briefly to consider
the ways that screens affect our physical health. Kids who
love gaming are hanging out with their friends online and
sitting for hours, a choice that's worse for weight and heart
health than an afternoon spent riding bikes together or
shooting hoops. Remind your kid of the real-life physical
activities that they enjoy, such as cycling, hiking, or walking
the dog, and brainstorm ways that they can make physical
activity a social event with friends so they're not sitting for
hours. Some parents have set house rules that require kids
to spend time outside for physical activity before they're
allowed to text or play games.

Pediatric orthopedists are also seeing a surge in neck
pain (sometimes called *text neck*) and neck and back injuries in kids that are caused by hours hunched over digital
devices. Thumb and wrist injuries are also increasingly

common as a result of texting. Encourage your children to take frequent breaks, to change positions when using digital devices, and to sit upright in a supportive chair instead of being hunched over on a bed or sofa. Suggest they occasionally text with their forefinger to ease repetitive stress injuries and to rest their hands by using the voice-to-text feature or actually calling on the phone.

Staring at screens also demands a lot of your child's eyes, causing eye fatigue, blurry vision, and dry eyes. Talk to your kids about the 20/20/20 rule, recommended by the American Optometric Association: look away from the screen every 20 minutes to focus on an object at least 20 feet away for at least 20 seconds. The AAP also recommends that children walk away from the screen for at least 10 minutes every hour. Timers can help to remind kids to look up periodically and walk away.

As we learn more about blue light, a wavelength given off by screens that can interfere with sleep when viewed at night, some parents wonder if they should consider getting their kids glasses that filter blue light; these are designed to block some blue light from reaching the eye during screen use. However, the American Academy of Ophthalmology (AAO) states there is a lack of evidence to support the use of the glasses. Instead, the AAO recommends switching off screens in the 2 to 3 hours before bed. The AAP suggests that all digital devices be gathered outside of the bedroom at night for charging at least 1 hour before bedtime to keep children and adults from frequently checking them because of FOMO.

How Screens Affect Our Kids' Ideas About Sex

Talking with kids about sex is difficult enough, but parents find themselves with the need to discuss the multitude of ways that sex intersects with digital devices. Kids have easy access to a range of sexualized content on their screens, from explicit music videos to a full video library of sexual acts on pornography sites. Research reveals that many kids encounter pornography online around age 13, although there are plenty of stories of kids stumbling across it earlier, sometimes accidentally.

I want to stress that interest in sex and seeking out information about it is normal and healthy. At the same time, there are some discussions among child development experts that online pornography may encourage kids to engage earlier in sexual activity and may contribute to unrealistic and unhealthy ideas about sexuality, gender roles, and expectations. Researchers who study young people's experiences with online pornography say it can portray unrealistic images of both men and women and encourage sexist attitudes and behaviors.

Online sexual content can be so unsettling and disturbing that it has prompted some parents to level with their tweens and teens. One mother, Tina, told her 12-year-old daughter that if she's ever curious about a word related to sex she should come to Tina first before searching for it online. She told me she'd rather just explain a sex act than have her daughter look it up and be misinformed.

Talking With Kids About Pornography

I believe that we as parents need to be smart and clear-eyed about the reality that our children will encounter pornography online and what the real effect of this content is on our children. This points to the importance of talking with kids early—as early as third grade—about the sexual content they may encounter online. Take a deep breath: This can be awkward, but it's important to be brave and do your best to muscle through the conversation. Laughing a little and letting your child know that this is a little difficult to discuss for you as well may help. I advise parents to think beyond 1 big conversation and to bring up the topic regularly and matter-of-factly. The following tips can help guide your conversation with your child:

Don't shame them. Do your best to keep shame and judgment out of the discussion. Let your child know that it's natural and normal to be curious about bodies and sex. If kids feel ashamed about their urge to seek out this content, they're less likely to come to you for help when they have questions.

Talk about what's problematic. Given the range of material available online, it's important to explain that the sexual content online can be disturbing and portrays an unrealistic view of bodies and sex. Let them know that pornography is fake and that real sex doesn't look or sound like what they see online. Such exposure can also complicate their romantic relationships in the future. Talk with older teens about the fact that the people in pornographic videos are often exploited. This may also be a good opportunity to speak about the larger topic of sex, the importance of waiting for the right time for sex and intimacy, birth control, and prevention of sexually transmitted infections.

Encourage questions. If you learn that your child has encountered sexual content online, ask them if they have any questions about what they saw. Take your cues from them, and try not to offer more information than they can handle or are developmentally ready for. If you are uncomfortable with this topic, you can reach out to your pediatrician for advice or to be a facilitator for the discussion.

Watch for signs of problematic pornography use. If teens stay up late and skip sleep to view online content, lock their bedroom doors, or leave a search history of pornographic sites, you may need to intervene. Ideally, you will want to be calm and matter-of-fact and say something like, "I notice that you've been visiting adult sites on the internet. I'd like to talk about some of the problems with these sites." Stories like Mason's (see the "The Importance of Explaining Sex" box) emphasize that kids need help understanding the world of pornography. I would encourage you not to let awkwardness or embarrassment prevent you from helping them figure it out.

THE IMPORTANCE OF EXPLAINING SEX

I was intrigued by a section in journalist Peggy Orenstein's book, *Boys and Sex*, in which she shares the conversations she had with a soft-spoken college student, "Mason" (name changed in the article). He reveals that he spent up to an hour a day watching pornographic videos in high school, even viewing them in the back seat of the car without his mom's knowledge while she drove him to the dentist. He recounts a time when his father found him watching pornography but did not comment much, except to say that he shouldn't watch it. Mason tells Orenstein that he wishes his dad had continued the conversation. He offers a suggestion of what it would have helped him to hear: "This will skew how you view women. It's not real. And it's not going to help you get a girl; it's only going to keep you from interacting with girls in a healthy manner." But his parents were too nervous to have those conversations. Notably, Mason eventually purchased himself a flip phone before college, in part to discourage himself from viewing pornography.

Sexting and Sexual Selfies

Based on what I hear from families, it's increasingly common for kids in middle school and high school to sext and send sexual selfies or provocative photos of themselves to others via the internet or their smartphone. Unfortunately, teens may not understand what can happen to those photos once they're sent or the legal consequences of sending or forwarding nude photos, especially for those under the age of consent. Talk with your child about resisting peer pressure to sext, and use resources about selfies, such as Common Sense Media, to launch the conversation, asking questions such as, "Have you seen this story?" "What did you think about it?" Often, kids have heard about sexting from peers already. You can also ask, "Has anyone at school talked about anything like this?" to help with the conversation.

BRANDON'S STORY

Brandon's mother confided in me that she'd just received a phone call from the parents of a girl in Brandon's class. Brandon and the girl were both freshmen in high school and had been texting racy photos of themselves to each other. When Brandon's mom checked his text thread, she was horrified; she had no idea her son even knew the terms he used in the text exchange. Fortunately, the girl's parents were on the same page as Brandon's; they were able to talk, commiserate a little, and even discuss each family's plan to stop the sexting. The incident highlighted that Brandon was further down the road in terms of sex and knowledge about it than his mom realized. She and her husband immediately increased their conversations with Brandon around sex and responsible technology use.

Making Mindful Decisions

I hope you feel empowered to make mindful decisions and to take healthy and productive actions about screen use for you and your family. The reality is that many adults and kids maintain unhealthy relationships with technology. I often think about the study in which researchers observed parents and kids interacting at a restaurant. If a scientist watched your family at the table, what would they see? Engaging with each other—or with digital devices?

It's important to notice our habits and regroup when we realize that we've fallen into unhealthy routines—it happens to all of us! Reevaluating how you and your kids use screens and developing a family media plan can help you reserve time for the healthier activities you value—and strengthen your connection to one another.

THE POSSIBILITY OF A FUTURE DRIVEN BY ARTIFICIAL INTELLIGENCE

Our technology is advancing at an exponential pace. Consider that Facebook has been available to most users only since 2006, and Google maps were first introduced in 2005, yet we cannot imagine our life without them. Similarly, the Blackberry, one of the very first smartphones, was born in the early 2000s, and we've become so dependent on this technology that most of us can't imagine not having our email, social media, online shopping, and texting right at our fingertips all the time. Futurists and experts predict that artificial intelligence will be the next big evolutionary step, leading to the automation of blue-collar jobs, as well as higher-skill positions in medicine and journalism. Scientists and technology experts are concerned about the effect on the future job market. In this future world, skills such as creativity, communication, and out-of-the-box thinking are likely to matter more to set us apart from artificial intelligence and keep us employed. To develop these talents, kids need free time to allow creative juices to flow and to make and recover from mistakes. In fact, many scientists report that brain breaks, including hobbies such as scuba diving and bread making, helped them to be more innovative.

Strategies for Being Screen Smart

To wrestle your family's attention away from digital devices and ensure that screen time isn't replacing healthy fundamentals such as physical activity and face-to-face connections, it's important to be thoughtful and proactive about screen use.

The following are a few strategies to consider:

Put down the devices yourself. Role modeling is essential. When I counsel families on issues such as better eating or physical fitness, the golden rule is to "say what you do, and do what you say." Kids watch what you do more than they listen to your words.

Make screen-free family time a habit. Designate times, such as mealtimes, when phones and tablets are turned off and put away. Plan 1 weeknight after 6:00 pm or part of the weekend, say Sunday mornings, when everyone agrees that they will not look at their devices.

"Just say no" to social media. Require kids to wait until they reach a certain age. Check out the Wait Until 8th campaign (https://www.waituntil8th.org) launched by parents who decided to delay their kids' phone use and social media engagement. It's important to place guardrails around how, when, and where kids use these technologies.

Resetting Our Relationship With Devices

A family media plan includes family goals and house rules around devices and social media. Think of this tool as a way to learn more about your child, including what they like about their digital experiences. View the media plan as a living, breathing document that you all revisit regularly and that can help strengthen the parent-child connection.

Use the following guidelines as you develop you own unique family media plan:

- **What locations and situations are screen-free zones in your home?** For example, I recommend prohibiting the use of devices at the dinner table. Make a family decision to turn off all devices 30 to 60 minutes before bed to help everyone wind down and improve sleep.
- **Where do devices get charged after bedtime?** To reduce the temptation for kids to text or check social media, many families place the devices in another room, such as the kitchen, to charge at night.
- **What types of content are OK for your child to use or view online?** Discuss what types of content require a parent's permission for them to use, and make sure everyone understands what content is off-limits.
- **What nonscreen activities does your family value?** Consider creating guidelines that reinforce values such as adequate sleep, reading, academics, connecting with family, and going outside. For example, maybe your family decides together that kids can't start texting or gaming until they've read a chapter, walked the dog, or called grandma or another family member. Another option is for them to earn screen privileges if all homework is done and they've scheduled 2 nonrelated screen activities with or without friends over the course of the week. Consider incorporating screen-free times (ie, 10:00 am to 11:00 am

on weekends) when no screens are allowed to be used. This will encourage the entire family to plan something fun or even relaxing during those times that involve no screens. This also allows children to think creatively.

Agree to revisit the media plan regularly, such as every 3 months, to decide what's working and what's not. I'll admit that these conversations can be daunting, especially if you know that your middle schooler will debate every limit you propose, but this effort is worth it. Treating kids respectfully and considering any reasonable suggestions they make seriously will increase the chances that they'll engage and that the discussion will be fruitful.

Remember, if you have any questions or concerns about your family and their digital media use, or about your children's physical and mental health, call your pediatrician. Pediatricians are wonderful resources on a variety of family issues and can provide consultation, mentoring, and coaching for parents, caregivers, children, and teens.

For more information, check out https://www.healthy children.org/English/media/Pages/default.aspx.

Toolbox Takeaways for Smart Digital Media Use

TAKEAWAY 1: **Access**

Make a bookmark on family computers that offers healthy, educational content about bodies and sex such as healthy-children.org, teenshealth.org, and commonsensemedia.org. Let kids know it's there. With access to this information, they may be less likely to use pornography as a way to satisfy their curiosity about sexual activity.

TAKEAWAY 2: **Alternatives**

Make a list of "insteads" that you hang on your fridge.
Turn to it when you or your child have the urge to pick up
a phone or tablet. Items might include making art, playing
a board game, taking the dog for a walk, throwing a ball
around, or listening to music.

TAKEAWAY 3: **Sharing**

Consider making car-pool time a no-screen time. Explain that
kids don't have to talk but announce a game or discussion topic
and encourage them to participate. Favorites include "Two
Truths and a Lie," in which kids list 3 statements and everyone
guesses which 1 is false. One mom I know asks her kids, "Who
laughed and who cried today?" to encourage sharing.

TAKEAWAY 4: **Fast**

Try a digital media fast with your whole family. It could be a
day long or for part of the day. This can allow creative time
but also potentially family activities such shooting hoops or
playing board games.

TAKEAWAY 5: **Engaging**

As long as it's appropriate, try the TikTok dances with your
kids. This may sound counterintuitive, but this is 1 way
to gain insight into what they are doing on social media
and keep the communication lines open—and get some
extra exercise! I recently tried a dance with my son, and he
became much more open and comfortable about sharing
what he and others were doing on social media. Remember,
open communication is an essential tool!

QUIZ

Is Your Child at Risk for Toxic Stress?

1. Does your child have at least 1 caring, responsive, consistent adult in their life?
    a. Yes. One or more nurturing adults have taken care of my child from birth. (0 points)
    b. Yes. My child has that now, but there were some periods when my child was in an inconsistent situation. (3 points)
    c. No. (5 points)

2. At night, how well does your child sleep?
    a. Soundly—if they get up to use the bathroom, they fall right back to sleep. (0 points)
    b. Pretty well, though they may wake up occasionally in the night and have trouble falling back asleep. (2 points)
    c. My child regularly has trouble sleeping, even when they are tired. They may experience frequent nightmares. (5 points)

3. How does your child deal with frustration, such as
   being told "no" or to turn off a video game?
   a. They can usually roll with it without a lot of
      drama. (0 points)
   b. They may respond on occasion with tears
      or a tantrum, but with a little guidance they
      usually recover quickly. (2 points)
   c. They respond on occasion with tears or a
      tantrum, and it takes work on my part to
      help them calm down. (4 points)
   d. It's meltdown city. My child is regularly
      prone to tears or angry outbursts when
      faced with roadblocks of any type. (5 points)

4. How often does your child show signs of anxiety?
   Common symptoms include rapid breathing, sweaty
   palms, trembling arms or legs, complaints of dizziness,
   headaches, stomachaches, digestive problems, or
   muscle pain in the jaw.
   a. My child doesn't show signs of anxiety.
      (0 points)
   b. My child sometimes shows signs of anxiety,
      usually in the lead-up to a stressful event,
      such as a big test or music recital. (2 points)
   c. My child is pretty anxious but has multiple
      tools that they use to address it, such as deep
      breathing, exercise, and sessions with a coun-
      selor or psychotherapist. (3 points)
   d. My child experiences these symptoms reg-
      ularly, at least a few times a week, and we
      have not figured out how to address it.
      (5 points)

5. How many traumatic events has your child experienced in their life? These may include being abused verbally, physically, emotionally, or sexually; having a parent with a substance use disorder; having an incarcerated parent; experiencing the separation or divorce of parents; being bullied; experiencing racism; or witnessing the abuse of a parent.

    a. None (0 points)

    b. 1 (2 points)

    c. 2 (4 points)

    d. 3 or more (5 points)

Add up your score. Total _____

What Your Score Means

0 to 8 points: Your child's stress levels appear to be low, which is good news. A little bit of stress is inevitable for kids, but 1 of your jobs as a parent is to help them cope with stress and to be attuned to the signs that stress has become too much for them. We explore those signs in this chapter and how best to manage them.

9 to 16 points: Stress is part of life, and it seems as if your child is feeling at least some negative effects of it. The good news is that researchers have found that several things—especially a supportive adult—can protect kids against the most serious consequences of stress.

17 to 25 points: Your child appears to be struggling with severe, prolonged stress. This increases their chances of experiencing serious, lifelong consequences. It's time to learn more about what's at stake and take some healthy steps to help your child get back on track and thrive.

CHAPTER 5

Understanding the Effects of Toxic Stress

've seen many families living highly stressful lives. After all, stressful circumstances are part of being human. Who hasn't faced a tough job or a layoff, a health problem, financial strain, or the death of a loved one? Even positive changes, such as learning to ride a bike or starting high school, can activate the stress response in children and teens, causing short-term spikes in stress hormone levels and heart rate.

A little bit of short-term stress is inevitable and may even benefit children by increasing their ability to be resilient and ensuring that they grow up healthy. More severe stress should be something a caregiver addresses to ensure it doesn't begin to affect their child for longer periods of time. When stress becomes particularly harmful, it is referred to as *toxic stress,* and it occurs when a child is exposed to severe stress repeatedly, sometimes over longer durations of time. When the body stays in this activated state for too long, it can take a negative toll on a child's mental and physical health, behavior, and ability to learn and focus.

The 3 Main Types of Stress

To help our children grow up to be healthy, functioning adults, we need to understand the basics of stress—what it is, how it affects a child's body, and how we can manage or even prevent it. Researchers who study stress on children classify it in 3 categories:

Positive stress. Sometimes events can trigger stress. Examples could be performing in a play, taking a test, or learning a new sport. Such events cause a brief elevation in heart rate and release of stress hormones, but they are for a brief interval as the symptoms abate and the systems soon return to homeostasis. This type of stress accompanies anything that might make a person feel uncomfortable but also allows growth of skills and mind. This type of stress is not usually a concern for long-term effects and is good for our kids to learn to be flexible and be OK with situations that may challenge them.

Tolerable stress. Difficult emotional events, such as the death of a beloved pet, a sudden hospital stay, or a scary car accident can lead to tolerable stress. If the event is time limited and the child has at least 1 supportive caregiver to help them cope with the stress, research shows that a child's body recovers quickly, without any lasting damage physically. If stress such as this is prolonged, though, or support is not present, it can have long-lasting effects.

Toxic stress. Toxic stress is very severe and often frequent. It can be the result of enduring experiences such as physical or emotional abuse, neglect by a parent, poverty, racial profiling, or having a family member who misuses drugs or alcohol. The damage of toxic stress can vary, depending on a child's genetic predisposition and the duration and intensity of the stressful experiences. Research shows that the presence of at least 1 responsive, supportive adult in a child's life may prevent and even counteract the effect of toxic stress. If children don't have the support of a loving, responsive adult to help buffer them from the effects of these experiences, the reoccurring stress can cause harm to their organs and immune system and even negatively affect brain development. Many different circumstances can lead to toxic stress for kids. When a situation creates unrelenting stress, and the child is left to cope with it without help, toxic stress can worsen. As a pediatrician, I've seen what toxic stress looks like, and I'm concerned by the research showing that it has alarming health consequences, sometimes lasting throughout a child's life into adulthood. This ripple effect can take a toll on physical health, mental health, and lifelong happiness.

Adverse Childhood Experiences (ACEs)

To understand toxic stress better, you may find it helpful to learn about ACEs (Figure 5.1), which stands for *adverse childhood experiences,* and refers to potentially traumatic events that can have a big effect on a child's health and well-being.

These experiences include physical, emotional, verbal, or sexual abuse as a child or neglect, a situation in which a child's needs for food, clothing, or love and affection are not met. It could include physical abuse to the child or even living in a situation where another person such as a mother is being physically or emotionally abused. Other common ACEs involve a family member with a substance use disorder who lives in the home, a family member who attempts or dies by suicide, an incarcerated parent, the separation or divorce of parents, mental illness in the home, a serious or life-threatening medical condition in the nuclear

FIGURE 5.1

What Are ACEs? And How Do They Relate to Toxic Stress?

WHAT ARE ACEs?
AND HOW DO THEY RELATE TO TOXIC STRESS?

"ACEs" stands for "Adverse Childhood Experiences." These experiences can include things like physical and emotional abuse, neglect, caregiver mental illness, and household violence.

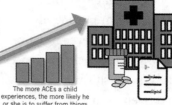

The more ACEs a child experiences, the more likely he or she is to suffer from things like heart disease and diabetes, poor academic achievement, and substance abuse later in life.

TOXIC STRESS EXPLAINS HOW ACEs "GET UNDER THE SKIN."

Experiencing many ACEs, as well as things like racism and community violence, without supportive adults, can cause what's known as toxic stress. This excessive activation of the stress-response system can lead to long-lasting wear-and-tear on the body and brain.

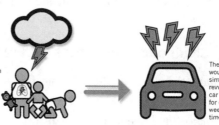

The effect would be similar to revving a car engine for days or weeks at a time.

WE CAN REDUCE THE EFFECTS OF ACEs AND TOXIC STRESS.

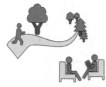

For those who have experienced ACEs, there are a range of possible responses that can help, including therapeutic sessions with mental health professionals, meditation, physical exercise, spending time in nature, and many others.

The ideal approach, however, is to *prevent* the need for these responses by reducing the sources of stress in people's lives. This can happen by helping to meet their basic needs or providing other services.

Likewise, fostering strong, responsive relationships between children and their caregivers, and helping children and adults build core life skills, can help to buffer a child from the effects of toxic stress.

ACEs affect people at all income and social levels, and can have serious, costly impact across the lifespan. **No one who's experienced significant adversity (or many ACEs) is irreparably damaged**, though we need to acknowledge trauma's effects on their lives. By reducing families' sources of stress, providing children and adults with responsive relationships, and strengthening the core life skills we all need to adapt and thrive, we can prevent and counteract lasting harm.

Center on the Developing Child 🛡 HARVARD UNIVERSITY

Learn more about ACEs from the Centers for Disease Control and Prevention.
For more information: https://developingchild.harvard.edu/ACEs

family, or witnessing the abuse of a parent. Bullying, poverty, and systemic problems such as racism are also considered ACEs. The more ACEs a child has experienced, the more likely they are to have health problems such as heart disease, diabetes, obesity, or depression at any time in life. ACEs are also linked with academic struggles and an increased risk of substance use or dependency.

ACEs can disrupt a child's sense of safety and increase their risk of developing toxic stress, in part because each experience moves the body's stress response to overdrive. According to an analogy from the Center on the Developing Child at Harvard University, ACEs are like revving a car engine for days or weeks at a time, causing a huge amount of wear and tear on the engine. Similarly, when a child's body is exposed over weeks and months or even years to a stress response, it also can experience a similar type of breakdown.

An estimated 2.7 million US children have an incarcerated parent. Studies show that these kids often have multiple adverse experiences: They may have lived with a parent with substance use problems or mental illness, for example, and family members who remain at home may struggle with financial trouble because of lost wages and costly legal fees. Children may also feel shame about their parent's prison time or lonely, scared, or angry and have little support from the adults who remain nearby. All of this has a real effect on the ways young brains and bodies develop.

Not every child responds in the same way to adverse events; their response depends on factors including their genetic predispositions, their age, and the kinds of support they receive from other adults in their lives. I cannot stress this enough: No matter how many ACEs a child has experienced, they are not damaged in an irreversible way. However, it is critical that we reduce the stress they face, provide caring support, and provide them skills to help them cope. Some of these skills are discussed in Chapter 1 and in various toolbox takeaways throughout the book. These include having nurturing, protective, and caring adults in a child's life; having a network or community that cares about the well-being of the child; and also having a circle of support for the parent. We also know that witnessing domestic violence between parents can affect the children, oftentimes influencing the way they view relationships and how they confront conflict and manage emotions. It can also influence their ability to cope with stress in their future, impair their self-worth, and make fostering future relationships difficult.

HOW COMMON ARE ACES?

ACEs can occur in any family. In a Centers for Disease Control and Prevention–Kaiser survey of adults in 25 states, roughly 61% of respondents indicated they had experienced at least 1 ACE in their lifetime, and nearly 1 in 6 reported they had experienced 4 or more types of ACEs. Research also shows that women and some racial and ethnic minority groups may be at greater risk for consequences on their mental and physical health when experiencing 4 or more ACEs.

How Toxic Stress Affects the Brain

During childhood, the brain undergoes critical development and experiences incredible growth in language, reading, and physical skills, as well as emotional growth. When stressed, bodies experience a rush of adrenaline, causing the heart rate to speed up and bodies to release a stress hormone called *cortisol*. The cortisol level drops if a child receives help from a parent or uses calming strategies such as exercise or meditation. But in cases of toxic stress, the body remains activated and on high alert, and the excessive cortisol can alter the way the brain develops. Parts of the brain that deal with emotions such as fear and anxiety may develop too many neural connections, while brain areas that affect reasoning, planning, and self-control may develop too few. This can change a child's stress response so that they respond to low-stress events as if they were full-blown emergencies. As a result, their stress response system activates more often and for longer periods. Studies show this can harm parts of the brain related to learning and memory and can also suppress a child's immune system, increasing their risk of developing conditions such as asthma, heart disease, diabetes, and other autoimmune diseases.

SEPARATION AT THE BORDER

It was incredibly alarming to see and hear about the children separated from their parents at the United States–Mexico border. Children of all ages were placed in frightening circumstances without a loving parent or guardian to soothe them and minimize stress. My colleagues and I continue to worry about the effects as these children grow; separating young children from their parents is similar to throwing a big rock into the pond of their developing brain. The ripples can last a very long time.

Warning Signs

Children experiencing toxic stress may seem anxious, cry frequently, have trouble sleeping, or lack an appetite. They may experience weight loss or gain or even hair loss. They can have symptoms that look a lot like attention-deficit/hyperactivity disorder. They may be aggressive or impulsive, have trouble focusing, or be hyperactive. Teens may have trouble keeping up with their academic studies and staying organized. They may have unexplained stomachaches or headaches or have frequent arguments and conflict with others.

I encourage parents to take all symptoms seriously and to consider possible sources of stress in their child's life. I can tell you from personal experience that stress can escalate and quickly become chronic and toxic for children—almost without you realizing it. Talk to your pediatrician if you are concerned about your child's health and well-being and request referrals to other sources of assistance such as a therapist.

My Story

When my daughter was in middle school and started experiencing anxiety, I took her to see a counselor. After a couple of appointments, the counselor explained that the tense verbal exchanges at home between me and my husband were triggering my daughter's anxiety. This was a startling wake-up call for both of us. We also noticed that our son over the past year had been frequently sick with migraines and stomachaches. That's when we knew we needed to do what we could to restore peace in our home.

After much deliberation and marriage counseling, my husband and I ultimately decided to move forward with a divorce. It was the hardest thing I've done in my life, but I realized that, in addition to other long-standing issues with our marriage, the chronic stress was terrible for my kids and was having significant ramifications on their mental and physical health. Now my ex-husband and I successfully co-parent, and regarding our situation, I feel grateful that we found a more harmonious, less stressful path forward.

Preventing or Dealing With Toxic Stress: What Parents Can Do

Learning and understanding toxic stress and its effects on children can be overwhelming, but there will always be reason for hope. Although toxic stress poses many real challenges, even children with a large number of ACEs can heal with the right kind of help. Acknowledging the full reality of toxic stress is the first step. The following important steps can help prevent and even heal toxic stress:

Remove sources of stress when possible. The first step is to remove your children from stressful circumstances as best as possible. If a family member's mental or physical illness is causing stress in the home, finding effective treatment can ease the strain for everyone. Also, talking about the treatment and what is being done to help the family member can open the lines of communication and provide children an opportunity to ask questions and share any concerns.

Prioritize the connection with your kid. Do the best you can to foster a strong relationship with your child. This may look different each day, but as long as the effort is there, that is what matters most. As we've discussed throughout this chapter, a strong relationship with at least 1 consistent adult can protect a child from the long-term damaging effects of toxic stress. Aim to be that person for your kid. You know best how your child typically responds to stressful circumstances. Can you provide ideas for coping that reflect what you know about them? For example, if your middle schooler becomes overwhelmed by large school projects, help them divide the project into smaller steps that feel more manageable.

Make your interactions age appropriate. Research shows that
a young child's brain develops best when parents use serve-
and-return strategies. When babies and toddlers babble,
cry, smile, or speak first words, parents respond with eye
contact, words, hugs, or other appropriate responses. Failing
to respond this way can be a form of neglect and a source
of stress for little ones, who need this warm, responsive
presence. As kids get older, research suggests that parental involvement may matter more to kids than the warm
responses. Consistently showing up at your teenager's sports
games or school concerts or being home in the evenings
even while they are busy with homework in their rooms may
feel important and supportive to them even if they don't
show it.

Get back to the basics. If your family is reeling from a traumatic experience or unprecedented stress in your lives, I
encourage you to revisit Chapter 1 and to consider some of
the healthy basics we discussed there, which can help buffer
against the effects of toxic stress. If you're still finding your
footing, start by adopting just 1 of the suggestions in that
chapter and take small steps, adding more when ready.

Play. Playful interactions and laughter can strengthen your
bond with your child and reduce stress levels for both of
you. Keep it simple; get outside to a nearby green space, trail,
or park for a short walk or bike ride. Watch a comedian or
silly movie that you both enjoy. Or play with your pets. If
you don't have your own dog or cat, borrow 1 from a friend
or neighbor.

Emphasize structure. Research shows that an organized,
structured home life helps to reduce the effect of stress on
adolescents. These structures can look different for each

family. You might plan a family pizza night on Fridays, a 5-minute check-in with you each day when your child gets home from school or even during the car ride home, or a nightly check-in at bedtime. Have your family pitch in with chores on Sunday afternoons, or advise that everyone be in the house for 90 minutes of screen-free time together on Wednesday evenings. Whatever you choose, the comfort of such routines can be expected and reassuring for all of you.

Consider counseling. If your child has faced multiple ACEs, they may benefit from the help of a psychotherapist or other mental health professional. If you're not sure where to find reliable help, check with your child's pediatrician, who can refer you to experts experienced in helping kids who have faced traumatic experiences. Don't let financial difficulties stop you; many skilled therapists accept insurance or provide services on a sliding scale basis.

Help your child set and achieve goals. Goal setting is an important life skill, and achieving goals can help kids feel calmer and more in control of their lives. Teach your child that the best goals are SMART.

- **Specific.** Goals such as, "I'm going to be the best basketball player at my school," are more difficult to achieve than a specific goal such as, "I'm going to improve my free-throw percentage."
- **Measurable.** Again, specificity helps. "I'm going to complete 100% of my assignments directly after school." A number can help your child see their progress. If your child has trouble with time management, then come up with an agreed-on number, such as 90%, so that they feel good about making and seeing their progress.

- **Attainable.** Help your child choose "Goldilocks goals" that aren't too easy or too challenging but feel just right for them.
- **Relevant/realistic.** The goal should feel important and beneficial to your child. Aiming for a full scholarship as a college gymnast might not happen for your child if they are not on the elite team by a certain age, but being skilled enough to compete on the high school team with their classmates might be possible—and fun.
- **Timely.** A concrete timeline makes goals more real, as in, "I'm going to train to finish that 5K race at the end of September."

Find help to cope with *your* stress. Easing some of your own burdens as a parent can help you to be a more responsive caregiver and support system. I'm a big fan of finding kind, like-minded parents for social activities, playgroups, and supporting one another. Friendship can be protective against stress. If you're in a crisis situation, do seek out people and organizations that can help. Your child's well-being depends on it.

Revisiting Positive Stress and Resilience

I don't want you to finish this chapter believing that it's your job as a parent to protect your child from *all* stress. Yes, it's important to know that major stress is a real problem with possible lifelong consequences. But as we considered at the start of this chapter, some forms of stress are positive, helping kids grow healthy and strong. And we *do* want our kids to learn ways to deal with adversity, to have the flexibility to cope with all that life throws their way, right?

After my divorce, my teen twins had many adjustments to make. They made the transition from eighth grade to high school, spent part of their time in 2 different homes, and had to adapt to a new version of life. At first it was very tough having mom and dad apart. While I provided plenty of emotional support and their dad did, too, we still experienced plenty of bumps in the road. These events were inconvenient but certainly not big emergencies. Learning to manage, cope, and bend with these changes, while knowing that they were deeply loved and connected to their parents, ultimately helped my children become more resilient and more responsible over the course of that first year. I feel strongly that these types of stressors helped them grow.

PANDEMIC LESSONS

When Mina's freshman year of college went virtual because of the COVID-19 pandemic, she became truly distressed. She had been looking forward to graduating from high school, moving out, making friends, and being invited to join a sorority. She sank into a depression in September, just barely attending her online classes.

Both her mom and her therapist engaged her in conversation about how she was not alone; many kids and families were in the same position. Her therapist suggested that Mina plan at least 1 social activity every day, even if it was just online get-togethers with a friend or family member for movie night or board games. She also began running and meeting a friend for tennis, a perfect socially distanced activity. Although it was very difficult, Mina slowly adjusted to this new way of life and in a few months started feeling a bit calmer. The loss of graduation and going to college as a freshman was a big loss, but she started realizing that she could learn to enjoy life in different ways and that life would eventually get better. The therapist pointed out that her disappointments were changes that offered her a chance to learn how to pivot more effectively, increase her resiliency in life, and adjust in the face of adversity.

Sometimes being a parent means allowing our kids to experience loss and pain. It's through these experiences that they become stronger and more resilient. In fact, children and teens who are exposed to some forms of adversity become more flexible in their thinking, too. They understand that everything will not always go as planned and can become more accepting of change.

One key way to help your child thrive is to be alert to stress and to ask yourself the following questions: Is a given situation a healthy challenge that will encourage my child to grow? Or is this a circumstance that poses the threat of toxic stress? If it's the latter, do you and your child have the support you need to get through this? Recognizing and taking stress seriously is 1 of the best ways to ensure your child has the tools needed to thrive.

Remember, it's never too late to make a change. The brain is capable of adapting and changing throughout life, and children who have faced adverse experiences will not automatically experience poor outcomes. Although recovering from toxic stress takes work, healing is possible, and the effort is worth it in the long run.

Toolbox Takeaways for Understanding the Effects of Toxic Stress

TAKEAWAY 1: Lean

Humans are communal creatures who do better when we cooperate and help each other. If you or your child is facing toxic stress, reach out to others for help.

TAKEAWAY 2: **Listen**

Check in with your child daily to find out how they're doing and what they're thinking and feeling. Listen attentively to their answers, which will help your child feel loved and understood. Listening is also a great way to check in on their stress levels.

TAKEAWAY 3: **Hope**

If toxic relationships are a source of stress for you or your child, it may be best for you to let go of these connections in favor of relationships that provide sustenance and hope.

TAKEAWAY 4: **Affection**

If your child is comfortable with physical affection (and it's important to follow their lead here), hugs and hand-holding can be an ideal way to ease stress. These actions help by triggering the release of oxytocin, a chemical that can reduce blood pressure and cortisol levels.

TAKEAWAY 5: **Connect**

Your child's relationship with you is the most important 1 in their life. As they grow, they also benefit from having other responsive adults in their lives, including teachers, coaches, and family and community members.

Does Your Family Prioritize Sleep?

1. On most nights last week, how many hours of sleep did your child or teen get?
   a. 7 hours or fewer (5 points)
   b. 8 hours (3 points)
   c. 9 or 10 hours (0 points)
   d. 11 hours or more (4 points)

2. Does your child or teen have a phone, tablet, or television in their bedroom?
   a. Yes, and the device is often turned on at night (5 points)
   b. Yes, but the device is switched off during sleep (3 points)
   c. No, all screens and devices are kept out of the bedroom. (0 points)

3. How often does your child seem tired or irritable or have trouble focusing during an average week?
   a. Every day (5 points)
   b. 3 or 4 days of the week (3 points)
   c. 1 day of the week (2 points)
   d. Pretty much never (0 points)

4. Does your child snore?*

    a. Yes, nightly (5 points)

    b. Yes, occasionally (2 points)

    c. No (0 points)

5. In an average week, how many days does your child get at least 30 minutes outside during daylight hours?

    a. Pretty much never (5 points)

    b. 1 or 2 days (4 points)

    c. 3 or 4 days (3 points)

    d. 5 or 6 days (1 point)

    e. Every day (0 points)

Add up your score. Total _____

*Note: Although snoring can be due to fatigue and exhaustion, it can also be a sign of sleep apnea or another underlying problem. If your child snores frequently, address it with your child's doctor.

What Your Score Means

0 to 5 points: Impressive! Your family is doing a great job prioritizing sleep and keeping your circadian rhythms strong, which benefits your child's mental, physical, and emotional well-being in many ways. Keep on making an effort to get those z's.

6 to 15 points: Your family has some strong sleep habits, but more can be done to get the full benefits of solid sleep (or make an effort to ensure that your child isn't getting too much). The right amount of sleep can help kids grow, boost their sports performance, increase their creativity and imagination, and help them succeed academically.

16 to 25 points: Your child is more than likely sleep-deprived, which makes it very difficult to cope. Take a hard look at family routines, sleep spaces, screen use, and more to help your child get more rest.

CHAPTER 6

Choosing Sleep as a Priority

As parents, most of us have experienced times of disrupted sleep, particularly when our children were babies. Think back to a night when you slept just 3 or 4 hours. How did you feel the next day? Were you able to focus on your work, or did you find it difficult to remember things and plan your day? Were you irritable at small things? And did you reach for a quick, unhealthy food option versus the healthy choice?

If sleep can have a huge effect on our well-being as adults, imagine the effect on our children. Very few children get the amount of sleep needed to thrive during the day. A survey from the Centers for Disease Control and Prevention showed that 6 of 10 middle schoolers and 7 of 10 of teenagers don't get the recommended amount of sleep. Failing to get quality sleep creates myriad problems beyond those based on a person's mood. Research shows that children who are sleep-deprived are at increased risk of developing conditions such as diabetes, obesity, and poor mental health, as well as behavior and attention issues.

Anna, a child I saw in my practice when she was 9 years old, was brought in by parents who were concerned about her inability to focus in the classroom. Anna was a very intelligent child, but her grades had dropped recently, and she often acted out in class. I asked Anna and her parents a few questions about her daily diet and about her quality of sleep. It turned out that even though bedtime was at 9:30 pm, she usually left her room for snacks, to use the bathroom, and to pack her backpack, pushing her bedtime later. She had to be up by 6:00 am to catch the school bus at 6:50 am, making most mornings a struggle. She often found herself running for the bus and skipping breakfast. I asked Anna to keep a diary of her sleep for a week. The diary revealed that she wasn't falling asleep most nights until 11:00 pm or even 11:30 pm, leading to fewer than 7 hours of sleep many nights. We discussed creating a pre-bed routine to help her relax and signal to her brain and body that it was time to sleep. I asked her to start the bedtime routine at 8:30 pm, with the goal of being in bed, lights out by 9:00 pm. And once the lights were out, Anna had to stay in bed. No more snacks, no more organizing her backpack, no more distractions. These strategies would help her prioritize and get better sleep on a nightly basis.

When I saw Anna 2 months later, she and her parents reported that it had taken a week to get the hang of the new routine, but Anna was now in bed on school nights by 9:00 pm. Anna still needed nightly coaxing to start the wind-down routine, but Anna's parents helped keep her accountable. They knew the new routine was working when Anna was up, ready for school, and fully fed before leaving for the bus. At school, Anna seemed much calmer, more cheerful, and more attentive in the classroom.

> ## HOW MUCH SLEEP DOES YOUR CHILD NEED?
>
> The National Sleep Foundation (NSF) recommends that children aged 6 to 13 get 9 to 11 hours of sleep a night. For teenagers aged 14 to 17, the NSF recommends 8 to 10 hours of sleep a night.

Insufficient sleep can cause attention issues that may look like attention-deficit/hyperactivity disorder (ADHD). With Anna, we looked into her getting more sleep before we looked into other possible causes of her focus issues. She was at least 2 hours short of the recommended amount of sleep for her age every night, which meant that over the course of just 5 days, she was losing out on the equivalent of an entire night's worth of sleep. No wonder she was having trouble concentrating!

The Current State of Sleep

Our bodies have evolved for the sleep-wake pattern, yet our routines today conflict with our internal clocks, says researcher Satchin Panda, PhD, who studies circadian rhythms, or the body's internal clock. We live and work indoors most of the time, using artificial light that's dimmer than the light outdoors, even on a cloudy day. In the evening, we continue peering at screens, including TVs, smartphones, computer monitors, and tablets, exposing our eyes and brains to blue light, a wavelength of light that makes us alert. That's just 1 of the reasons that it can be difficult to fall asleep and get the restful sleep we need.

Being mindful of daylight would be 1 way to reincorporate those long-forgotten healthy habits. Simply walking outside for 10 to 15 minutes once or twice a day can help reset our clock by exposing our retinas (the back of our eyes) to sunlight. Additionally, it is essential to shut down our devices optimally about 1 hour before we go to bed. This protects us from the blue light that can interfere with our sleep cycle and helps maintain melatonin levels that help us with sleep. In the spring and summer, we can align more of our activities with our circadian clock by waking up closer to daybreak and winding down most thinking processes and energetic activities by sunset. Although this may not be practical all the time, it's helpful to know that the closer we are to our natural rhythms, which follow daylight and nighttime, the better the effects on our bodies are for optimal health.

Caffeine and Your Teen

Another factor that affects sleep is caffeine. My teenage patients often tell me that they love coffee. One young teen I know visits a local coffee shop with a group of friends almost every day after school, where they order lattes and other blended coffee drinks. He pointed out that he always orders the decaf version, but this 4:00 pm habit is still worrisome. Coffee beverages are loaded with calories and sugar, which don't help efforts to maintain a healthy weight, and "decaffeinated" does not mean "caffeine free." Even decaf coffee contains *some* caffeine. A little bit of this stimulant chemical may be OK for some children, but others may be more sensitive to it. We all have different bodies and different food sensitivities. And even kids who don't seem sensitive can experience sleep disruption if they consume caffeine in the late afternoon. As sleep researcher Matthew Walker, PhD, explains, if an adult has a cup of coffee at 2:00 pm, a quarter of the caffeine is still in the brain at midnight. Even if that adult falls asleep, the caffeine in their brain can decrease the amount of deep, non-rapid eye movement (REM) sleep they get. And that's the phase of sleep that's especially restorative.

An alternative way to be awake—or stay awake—can be to exercise. Even a 10-minute jog outside or dancing to music can help your teen stay energized and focused on the next round of homework or studying. This is a great way to get an energy boost. Also, dehydration can often lead to feeling tired. It's amazing how much drinking enough water can make a difference in our hourly to daily energy levels. Encourage everyone in your family to drink at least 6 to 8 glasses of water a day.

Procrastination and Your Teen

Another sleep stealer is the habit that researchers call *bedtime procrastination*. Kids (and parents too) tend to put off sleep by watching 1 more show or checking social media and scrolling mindlessly, eventually crawling into bed later than intended. Blue light from screens can interfere with sleep, so avoid devices 30 minutes to an hour before attempting to fall sleep. Realistically, our teens might need to complete homework by using their computers until late, and those will be the days that you may have to excuse them from this rule. But in general, trying your best to implement this rule will be more beneficial in the long run. Completing homework after school or directly after dinner can help avoid late-night homework fests.

Many elementary school kids become drowsy and feel ready to sleep between 8:00 and 9:00 pm. But as they grow older and enter the teenage years, they undergo a sleep phase delay, which shifts drowsiness to a later time, usually between 10:00 and 11:00 pm. Despite this change, they still need an average of 9 hours of sleep a night, making a 7:15 am school start time a large issue for high schoolers. Teens who fall asleep around 11:00 pm but have to wake up around 6:00 am to arrive at school on time may be getting only 7 hours of sleep per night. By the end of the week, they're exhausted. The American Academy of Sleep Medicine and the American Academy of Pediatrics have both issued position statements calling on middle schools and high schools to delay start times until 8:30 am or later to allow children and teens more time for the sleep they need. To treat the sleep debt, I allow my own children to sleep in on weekends and holidays till 10:00 or even 11:00 am. At the very least, it can help them get the quality of sleep they need and refresh them.

This is 1 of those situations that I believe parents can potentially influence by becoming active with their schools. Parent Teacher Associations are great for this because they give parents a voice. Individual parent-teacher conferences are invaluable because teachers not only share academic information but also can identify other areas of importance for your child, including social and emotional well-being and executive functioning.

How Sleep Deprivation Physically Affects Our Children

Kids who don't get enough sleep on a regular basis may face health consequences. Lack of sleep has been associated with an increased risk of developing obesity. One recent study found that preschoolers who regularly stayed up past 9:00 pm were more likely to be overweight once they reached school age. The researchers noted that their study didn't prove that lack of sleep *causes* children to gain weight. However, late bedtimes could be a sign of an irregular life in which kids ate late at night and gained excess weight, for example.

Other studies have shown that loss of sleep changes the body's hormones, suppressing the hormone that halts overeating and elevating the hormone that makes us hungry, which can make children more likely to eat big portions and more snacks when they're tired. Another small study found that teen boys who were obese and were placed on a diet lost more weight when they began a personalized sleep plan that helped them get 1.2 hours of extra sleep per night.

People who are regularly short on sleep face an increased risk of developing prediabetes and type 2 diabetes. Early research shows that chronic sleep deprivation may weaken the immune system, making the body more prone to infections and viruses. Tired kids are also more likely to be injured, possibly because fatigue impairs motor skills and slows reaction times. Drowsiness is a big factor in car accidents; about 1 in 10 crashes are due to drowsy driving, and young people between the ages of 16 and 24 cause more than 50% of them. One study found that teens who sacrificed sleep were more likely to engage in risky behaviors, such as not wearing a helmet while riding a bike, texting while driving, or riding in a car driven by someone who has been drinking. The study also suggested that insufficient sleep might may lead teenagers to ignore the possibility of negative consequences—though they point out that depression in teens could contribute to sleep issues and cause them to take unnecessary risks.

Lack of sleep can worsen symptoms for children who have ADHD. If your child has ADHD, check your child's medication prescription with their doctor. A different dose or a different schedule of taking the medicine can help lessen interference with sleep. Sometimes switching a medication to another alternative can help as well. Talk with your child's doctor if you suspect the medicine is causing a problem. Lastly, if your kid has ADHD, stick to a structured schedule. A set bedtime with a bedtime routine, physical activity, and even a set wake-up time will help to encourage and maintain better sleep habits and sleep duration.

SLEEP AND ITS EFFECT ON MOOD AND MENTAL HEALTH

It's also important for parents to understand how a lack of sleep can take a toll on a child's mental health. A recent study found that poor sleep quality was linked to depression, anxiety, impulsive behavior, and poor cognitive performance. Children 9 to 11 years old who slept for fewer than 7 hours a night were 53% more likely to have behavior problems.

This is not surprising when you consider the effects on adults as well. When 1,000 adults with sleep issues were followed for 3 years and compared with those who did not have insomnia, those with sleep disturbances were more likely to develop depression. Additionally, those with sleep issues who were depressed didn't respond to treatment as well as the ones who slept well.

The Benefits of Sleep

I often say that sleep is the unsung hero for helping our bodies and minds. In our fast-paced lives, it is so easy to let sleep fall to the wayside. But resting is vital for our health. The following are some of the great benefits of prioritizing sleep:

Reduces stress. A 2019 study of nearly 50,000 children found that children and teens who got at least 9 hours of sleep (the amount that researchers considered sufficient sleep) were the most likely to show signs of flourishing such as increased interest and curiosity in learning new things, completing homework, doing well academically, and finishing tasks that they started.

Increases learning. As we sleep, the brain stores information and memories from the day, forming new neural pathways that allow us to learn new things. Quality sleep makes us more creative. We dream during deep, REM sleep, and sleep scientists believe the brain often uses the time to work out problems. There are many stories of people who woke up with new ideas and solutions to problems. Beatle Paul McCartney has said that he came up with the tune for "Yesterday," golfer Jack Nicklaus once explained that he corrected his golf grip, and writer Mary Shelley had the inspiration for the book *Frankenstein*—all in their dreams. Sleeping on it apparently can yield breakthroughs. One way that I have had my kids comply with sleep habits is to talk with them frequently about the benefits of sleep but also, if they are cranky or unproductive, to ask them what time they went to bed and what time they woke up. These constant reminder conversations have helped them understand how sleep affects them. And, of course, I try to model the behavior I expect from them by following the same sleep strategies and habits myself.

CLEANING THE BRAIN

In recent decades, researchers have discovered the glymphatic system, a sort of sewage system in the brain that operates in high gear while we're asleep, washing away toxic proteins that have built up in the brain during waking hours. If we're short on sleep, and that deep brain wash can't occur, some of those wastes, beta-amyloid proteins, accumulate in the brain. A buildup of beta-amyloid proteins is linked to impaired brain function and Alzheimer disease.

Assists in physical growth. Sleep is also important for a child's physical growth. Children's bodies do much of their growing as they snooze because the secretions of the human growth hormone peak throughout the night.

Improves athletic performance. Sufficient sleep improves athletic performance, in part by improving coordination and giving stressed muscles and other tissues time to heal. Research shows that the less athletes sleep, the more likely they are to be injured. Explaining to children and teens that quality sleep can help them grow, boost their sports performance, aid in creativity, and increase emotional and academic success could motivate them to understand sleep better and learn to prioritize it more.

When kids are stressed out for various reasons, there are tools that can help calm them, activate the para-sympathetic system (the system that balances out the sympathetic fight-or-flight response system), and allow them to fall sleep.

- **Deep breathing.** Slowly take a deep breath while counting to 7, hold it for 5 seconds, and let go to relax the mind and muscles.
- **Talking.** Sharing their stress with a parent or another trusted friend or adult can help kids express what they are feeling.
- **Visualizing.** Thinking about a place where they feel happy and going to that place in their mind can help relax them and put them in a better frame of mind.

The Importance of Circadian Rhythms

Researchers have found that almost all cells and organs in our bodies have so-called clocks that determine what time of day they work best. Ignoring those natural rhythms can cause our physical and mental health to suffer in many ways. Satchin Panda, a circadian rhythm researcher, offers several tips for strengthening and synchronizing circadian rhythms for better sleep and overall health.

Make an outdoor habit. Getting outside every day for at least 30 minutes of daylight does wonders. The exposure to sunlight strengthens circadian rhythms and boosts alertness and mood, creating another reason to transition kids off their screens and into the great outdoors. You might also make outside time a family ritual by walking together during some mornings, or after dinner, no matter what the weather. Fun rain gear might help entice kids to head outside, even when it's wet.

Reduce screen time. Screens are a prime culprit in disrupting circadian rhythms. Panda's research found that the blue light emitted by smartphones, laptops, tablets, and other screens activates a protein in the eyes known as *melanopsin*, which reduces the body's production of melatonin, the hormone that makes us drowsy in preparation for sleep. Many studies show that the more screen time kids engage in, the less time they spend sleeping, partially because of the blue light the screens emit. Because blue light is activating, it's essential to limit screen time as bedtime nears. Many digital devices such as smartphones and tablets now come with a night mode that turns on after sunset, turning the screen yellowish and minimizing the amount of blue light they emit. As discussed in an earlier chapter, there are also glasses designed for screen use that filter blue light to block some of it from reaching the eyes. Some parents wonder if this is an option to help kids sleep better, but the American Academy of Ophthalmology states there is a lack of evidence to support use of the glasses. Instead, the American Academy of Ophthalmology recommends switching off screens in the 2 to 3 hours before bed.

Given the negative effects of blue light on sleep, it's important for families to make bedrooms a screen-free zone. That means no TV, tablets, or phones. It's best to be strict about this, given the necessity of quality sleep for kids. (Some parents hate to be the bad guy, but if they purchased their child's phone, they have a say over its use). If your child uses a phone alarm to wake up in the morning, opt for a separate alarm clock instead so the phone can be turned off. Kids should not be able to see the glowing screen in the night or have their sleep disrupted by the pings and buzzes of text messages or other alerts.

Limit the hours you eat. Panda's circadian rhythm research shows that the time of day we eat can affect how well we sleep. Eating gives your body the signal that it's daytime, interfering with the release of melatonin, the hormone that promotes sleep. Panda recommends that people eat their last meal of the day 2 to 3 hours before their target bedtime, which eliminates late-night snacking. This is a practice known as *time-restricted eating,* which is related to intermittent fasting and championed by many physicians and researchers for reducing the risks of heart disease, obesity, and diabetes. You might declare a new family rule— that the kitchen is closed at 8:00 pm every day. After all, a home is not a restaurant! And apart from the sleep benefits, halting after-dinner snacks is a smart way to help family members maintain a healthy weight. Some people may not do well with intermittent fasting or time-restricted eating, so talk to your pediatrician to see if this is a good idea for your family.

What Are Chronotypes?

As research has evolved in understanding our own internal clocks, we also have a better understanding of how different people may have differing circadian rhythms or *chronotypes*. Chronotypes are natural tendencies to be sleepy at a certain time and being wakeful at others; this might dictate how a person has an inclination to be a "night owl" or an "early bird." This can affect your best time to work, when you have the most energy, and even the best biological time to eat. Chronotypes are often based on several factors such as genes, age, and environment. Scientists feel that it is difficult to fight against these natural body tendencies, and it is beneficial to align with them if possible.

Dr Michael Breus, a clinical psychologist and widely known as "The Sleep Doctor," describes 4 chronotypes: the lion, who wakes up early and is most productive in the morning; the bear, who tends to follow the sunrise and sunset; the wolf, who tends to stay alert till late at night; and the dolphin, who is somewhat alert even when sleeping.

It's a good idea to understand your own chronotype, as well as your kid's type. My daughter tends to be productive in the morning with her schoolwork, while my son seems to get his best work done in the evening. Knowing this about your kids can help you tailor bedtimes more and avoid battles against the biological clock.

When Children Have Trouble Sleeping

If your child says they're not sleeping well on a consistent basis, or they regularly seem exhausted, it's important to check in with their pediatrician. Some kids may have an underlying medical issue that can prevent restful sleep. One of those conditions is obstructive sleep apnea. This occurs when the tissue in the back of the throat relaxes during sleep, preventing air from reaching the lungs and triggering a pause in breathing. These pauses can happen a few times a night or repeatedly, hundreds of times a night. Each pause causes the child to wake briefly, disturbing their sleep and making them very tired the next day. Typically, you can hear the person with this condition snoring, which becomes louder and then suddenly stops. This can be a potentially serious condition, affecting the heart and breathing. If you suspect your child or teen has this, talk to your pediatrician.

Mental health problems such as depression can also disrupt sleep. And sometimes medications, including those for ADHD and asthma, can disrupt sleep. Ask your child's pediatrician to look into and determine if this might be the case for your child. If your child shares that they're lying awake at night, unable to sleep, help them talk through what's going on. For example, are their anxious thoughts interfering with sleep? Some children sleep better if they jot down their concerns and anxieties in a notebook before bed, unloading them for sleep. Is it too hot in their bedroom? If so, they may need lighter pajamas or bedding. Sleep physicians tell patients who are unable to sleep to get out of bed after 15 minutes of wakefulness and start a quiet, even boring activity in another dimly lit room. Screens are not recommended in this situation because they activate the brain, while reading a less-than-exciting book or listening to instrumental music are 2 great options to encourage sleepiness. Changing locations prevents teens from associating their bed with sleeplessness, and keeping the lights low promotes drowsiness. Once they start feeling sleepy, they should head back to bed.

LIMIT NAPPING

Overtired children and teens might be tempted to nap after school; if they do this, encourage them to keep naps to less than an hour and to limit how often they nap. Longer naps and snoozing late in the day can interfere with nighttime sleep. Sometimes a power nap before dinner and before homework may help boost the energy level after a long day of school and activities, but it's generally not recommended after dinner because it may keep your child up later or cause sleeplessness. On weekends, make sure your kids are up well before late afternoon. If your child complains that they're drowsy later in the day, encourage them to go outside to shoot hoops, go for a walk or run, or take the dog out. If going outside is not an option, turn on some music and dance. For older teens, consider the many short workouts available online—maybe even do the workout with them!

Sleep Hygiene Habits for the Best Sleep

The term *sleep hygiene* suggests that sleep is just as important to good health as washing your hands and brushing your teeth. If your child is 1 of the more than half of US kids who doesn't get enough sleep, it's never too late to take steps to improve their sleep hygiene.

Create routine. To set the stage for quality, restorative sleep, help your child develop a calming routine that they repeat every night in the 15 to 30 minutes before bed. The routine signals to their brain and body that it's time to unwind. This might include taking a short shower, brushing teeth, dimming bright lights, and then reading for 10 minutes before lights out. Some kids like to take a few deep breaths, listen to soothing music, or say a prayer before they sleep. I know a 9-year-old whose mom reads him 1 chapter of a book they love before bed and an 11-year-old who jots down things she's grateful for in a notebook she keeps on her nightstand, which is a nice way to end the day on a positive note. Whatever makes sense and works for your child, try not to let the presleep routine become too elaborate; simplicity will make it easier to complete every night and will prevent kids from using it as a delaying tactic. It's important to build in time for this pre-bed routine. If your child's bedtime is 9:00 pm, help them start the routine at 8:30 pm so that they're ready to switch the lights off on time.

Do not allow screen time. Of course, this point bears repeating: Require your child to place phones and tablets outside the bedroom before they crawl into bed. This prevents them from seeing stimulating blue light at night, being tempted to scroll online or on social media into the wee hours of the night, or having their sleep disrupted by alerts. The American Academy of Pediatrics recommends keeping a TV out of your kid's bedroom, so consider removing it or ensure that your child knows not to use the TV to fall asleep.

Be cool. Sleep research reveals that people sleep best in a cool room around 65°F. This might sound chilly, but cooler temperatures make us drowsy and promote sleep. In fact, the body's temperature continues dropping through the night until about 5:00 am, when it starts to rise again. Some forms of insomnia are linked to issues with regulating body temperature. If your child complains that they're having trouble falling asleep, check to make sure that they're not using too many blankets or wearing heavy pajamas. One mom shared with me that when her kids have trouble falling asleep, she tells them to stick a hand or foot out from under the blankets. She's found that it cools them off and helps them fall asleep sooner.

Dim the lights. Bright light at night is stimulating, whereas nighttime darkness sends a message to the body that it's time to sleep. Use lamps with dim, incandescent bulbs or red bulbs (2 types of light that promote sleep) on the bedside table. Once lights are out, keep the bedroom as dark as possible to foster good sleep. Encourage your child to sleep without a night-light and consider light-blocking window shades to prevent any outside light from entering the bedroom.

Model the way. A key way to improve your child's sleep is to show them that restorative sleep is a priority *for you* as their parent. It's hard to convince them that sleep matters if they see you cleaning the kitchen or working on your computer at 11:00 pm (or later). Make it a goal to give sleep a higher priority than other activities after 9:00 pm. Try not to let pride about your lack of sleep creep into conversation with your kids. Don't let them hear you say things such as, "I'll sleep when I'm dead." They may not understand the joke or sarcasm and won't prioritize their sleep the way they should.

Say no. Be strict about saying no to at least some of the activities that will prevent you and your child from prioritizing sleeping. As parents, we have an important role in preparing our children for life on their own someday. As we help them prepare for college and beyond, we teach them how to do laundry and manage their time, and we educate them on the basics of good nutrition, but prioritizing sleep is just as important to their emotional and physical well-being.

Toolbox Takeaways for Prioritizing Sleep

TAKEAWAY 1: **Conversations**

Talk about the importance of sleep and its positive effects often. I found that the more often I explained this to my own kids, the more it stuck in their heads. Having frequent conversations about why it's a priority can lead to children not only understanding but also making it a priority.

TAKEAWAY 2: **Rules**

Plan *how* to prioritize sleep with your kids. Should there be a rule about sleepovers? One of the rules I always advocate is to say no to sleepovers unless they occur on a long weekend or during holidays. One night of little sleep can roll into a whole week of late starts and attention issues in school. Talk to your kids about rules around conserving sleep.

TAKEAWAY 3: **Reinforcement**

If your child has had a good night of sleep, point out and acknowledge the specific steps they took to prioritize their sleep. Reinforcing good habits can go a long way.

TAKEAWAY 4: **Transparency**

Remember, especially on weekdays, to go to sleep on time. This means letting your kids know that you are settling your body and mind. This could include reading, a few minutes of deep breathing, or listening to soft music. Whatever you decide to do, let your children know your plan.

TAKEAWAY 5: **Relaxation**

Offer your children tips on what to do if anxiety keeps them from falling asleep or if they wake up during the night. A big test or an argument with a friend could make their mind spin in circles. Advise them to take 6 deep breaths, slowly counting backward from 100. If that doesn't work, they can try reading for 5 minutes. Even 3 minutes of mindfulness meditation can calm the mind and help them to feel sleepy.

QUIZ

Parents: Do You Have a Handle on Your Stress?

1. How would you describe your current stress levels?
   a. Not bad—my life may be hectic at times, but it's balanced with rest and fun, and I feel calm and able to cope most of the time. (1 point)
   b. I really feel the effects of stress sometimes. If I'm honest, it's probably too often, but I do have healthy strategies I can use to get myself back to equanimity. (3 points)
   c. Emotional distress is a daily reality for me. My body often feels tense and unwell, and I'm regularly overwhelmed or anxious or feel down. (5 points)

2. How often do you engage in some kind of physical exercise?
   a. Most days of the week I take a walk, a run, a bike ride, a swim, a fitness class, or some other form of movement. (0 points)
   b. I manage to exercise 2 or 3 times a week. (2 points)

    c. I usually walk or do some form of physical activity at least once a week. (4 points)

    d. Physical activity isn't really part of my life. (5 points)

3. Describe your social network.

    a. I have a decent group of close friends and loved ones, as well as coworkers, neighbors, and acquaintances from different areas of my life. I have people around me I can count on. (0 points)

    b. I am very close to a few friends and/or family members. We have connected, loving relationships, but I'm not especially social otherwise. (2 points)

    c. I have family and friends I think I could count on in an emergency, though I'm not sure. (4 points)

    d. Right now I don't have a lot of close relationships. (5 points)

4. How many days on average per week do you get 7 or 8 hours of sleep at night?

    a. 7 days (0 points)

    b. 6 days (1 point)

    c. 4 or 5 days (2 points)

    d. 2 or 3 days (3 points)

    e. Maybe once (4 points)

    f. Never (5 points)

5. How often do you participate in activities you would describe as fun, either by yourself or with others?

      a. Every day, without fail (0 points)

      b. A couple times a week (1 point)

      c. Once a week (3 points)

      d. Maybe once or twice a month (4 points)

      e. Fun? I can't remember the last time that happened. (5 points)

Add up your score. Total _____

What Your Score Means

0 to 5 points: You're impressively stress resilient, thanks to your healthy habits, and that likely benefits your family. Make an effort to stick with this wise lifestyle. And be mindful of the ways that negative stress can creep up and knock you off your stride.

6 to 15 points: Your stress levels ebb and flow, and sometimes the stress becomes too much. In those moments, you often know what it takes to feel better, though it's sometimes tough to restart those habits. This chapter offers a lot of strategies to help you—and your family—get back on track and stay there.

16 to 25 points: Stress is causing you to struggle. It's time to pause and reflect on what needs to change so you feel calmer, healthier, and more resilient. You are worth the effort. And when you're in a good place, the rest of your family benefits.

CHAPTER 7

Replenishing the Cup for the Stressed-out, Overwhelmed Parent

As we speak about our quest to raise children who are happy and healthy and who can manage stress well, we've discussed many essential fundamentals that need to be made priorities, including food, sleep, and emotional wellness. But there is 1 key concept that we must also delve into as well, and that is the health of *you*, the parent or caregiver. There is an old saying about filling your own cup before you can fill another's. This is true of us as parents: How can we keep on giving our time and energy, even with our most heartfelt intentions, and expect the best if we run on empty? It is very important to acknowledge our own role and our own physical and mental health to make parenting a success.

In the last few decades, society's expectations of parents have increased. Parents are often expected to take on after-hours and weekend tasks answering emails and managing projects. In a recent survey, nearly two-thirds of parents stated parenting seemed harder today than what they perceived it was like 20 years ago, citing modern reasons such as screens, the rise of social media, technology, violence on TV, and increasing expenses. Parents are often pulled in many directions, and many feel that their relationships suffer and that they sacrifice time for themselves.

In this chapter, we turn the spotlight on us as parents. With a healthy dose of love and self-compassion, I touch on the stresses we face and how we can cope without losing our sanity or dissolving into a puddle of guilt. How can we find joy in the daily hustle? It's important to pace ourselves, and, when possible, to find meaning along the way.

Part of our job as parents is to think about how our choices affect our children. As our child's main role model, we can't expect them to learn to lead a healthy, balanced life if we aren't making healthy choices ourselves.

The Parental Pressure to Do It All

Whether you are a mom, a grandma, a dad, or an aunt taking care of kids, we all feel the need to be patient and nurturing with our kids, take them to whatever activities they are in, and throw them a celebratory birthday party, as well as be a loving partner or daughter or son. We feel the pressure to succeed at our careers while trying to maintain a comfortable home that mirrors what you may see on TV or social media. Many of us almost always say yes when asked to volunteer or help out with a school event.

The anger and frustration we can feel while juggling parenting with all of life's other demands is understandable. But it requires healthy outlets. These outlets are important for our own well-being and the well-being and safety of our kids. Many parents may admit to scolding their child or feeling angrier than they should when already feeling frustrated. As clinical psychologist Laura Markham, PhD, author of *Peaceful Parent, Happy Kids: How to Stop Yelling and Start Connecting,* explained on the WebMD Health Now podcast, "It's hard to remain emotionally generous with your child when you're running on empty. And what do children need from us? They need emotional generosity." But just how *do* we refill our tank? How do we find that emotional generosity?

Self-care Fundamentals for Parents

Staying sane and providing our children the nurturing they need starts with taking care of ourselves. This requires a few baseline habits. As we discussed in Chapter 2, all kids need a set of fundamentals—sleep, food, water, and exercise—to be healthy and strong. It's no surprise that those same basics are essential for adults.

The challenge for parents is to stop viewing these basics as luxuries and to see them as nonnegotiable priorities. It also important to be kind to yourself. We've all had the experience of being busy and temporarily falling off the wagon with good habits. The important thing is to pick yourself back up lovingly and start again with the healthy choices the next day, without beating yourself up.

The Physical and Emotional Toll of Stress

We all know that chronic stress can feel miserable. It's no surprise that it takes a toll on your health. Stress can cause headaches and migraines, interfere with sleep, and even weaken immunity. Acute, short-term stress can trigger vomiting and diarrhea, and long-term stress is linked to irritable bowel syndrome. Notably, women experience irritable bowel syndrome twice as often as men. Women under stress may also experience more severe premenstrual syndrome symptoms and have a lower sex drive.

Chronic stress can also raise blood pressure and heart rate. Long-term stress increases the risk of anxiety and depression, possibly because it exposes the body to overly high levels of the brain chemical cortisol. And research shows that women who are stressed are more likely than men to develop anxiety and depression. Multiple studies show that stress negatively affects romantic relationships as well. One study found that when couples both had a stressful experience, they were less likely to offer hugs or supportive words to each other. Male partners were particularly likely to limit their support when the female partner responded to stress with strong emotions.

Our stress also affects our kids. Children and teens *know* when we are stressed, upset, or angry, and this can manifest itself by making them stressed out, too. It's similar to a healthy diet. We can't expect our children to make healthy food choices when we pick unhealthy foods ourselves. Similarly, if we want our children to be calm and resilient, we ourselves need to be able to manage and cope well with stress.

Sleep

Adults need 7 to 9 hours every night, according to the National Sleep Foundation. Lack of sleep not only makes it difficult to stay focused during the day but also harms your brain health. Getting enough sleep as a parent is difficult. We manage the to-do list, often bringing it to bed with us. A 2018 study found that people who are even a little short on sleep tend to avoid interactions with others. In another study, researchers found that college students who reported better sleep were more empathetic toward others. When you're foggy and irritable, it's hard to cut your partner some slack when they forget to do something, or it may be more difficult to listen carefully when they need someone to talk or vent to. It's difficult to resolve a disagreement or laugh together when you're feeling pushed to the limit. It makes sense that communication is stronger when both partners are rested enough to be patient and focused and have the mental space to give each other the benefit of the doubt.

I have had many times when I can't fall asleep or have woken up in the middle of the night. When my son was regularly becoming sick and missing school, or there were layoffs at my work, I became very worried. Additionally, at bedtime, I had the urge to tackle 1 more email or look at social media to relieve my anxiety. But over time, I found that this worsened my likelihood of falling sleep and staying asleep. So I started focusing on my sleep hygiene. This involved making a mental note of when I wanted to go to bed so I could get 7 hours of restful sleep and then backtracking to the best time to shut down my laptop and restrict my phone use. I bought a couple of books and placed them on my bedside table, and I bought giant fluffy pillows for the bed. On most nights, my current routine is to climb into bed and try to read for at least 10 to 15 minutes, which helps me to calm down, feel drowsy, and fall sleep.

Sometimes putting away the smartphones or electronic devices is easier said than done. Many of us are answering emails or engaging in a little bit more of the social media buzz. We know that these digital sleep stealers emit activating, sleep-disrupting blue light (as we talked about in Chapter 6) that can halt your body's production of melatonin, the hormone that triggers drowsiness. Some ways to counteract this is to set a mini schedule for yourself with strict screen use rules. I have had success with the following relaxation habits:

- **Set a pre-bed routine.** This helps you start to wind down in the evening. Know what time you need to wake up, and make sure that your bedtime is 7 hours prior to that. It helps me to give myself 1 last screen check-in, about 45 minutes before I intend to go to sleep, and then I put on the "do not disturb" feature. When I can, I place the phone as far away from the bed as possible. (Bonus—placing the phone far from the bed can also help you to get up when the alarm goes off and refrain from continually hitting the snooze button!)
- **Read before bed.** Keep a book or 2 on your coffee table or bedside table. It seems basic, but it works wonders to put my mind at rest before sleep. I recommend reading for

about 20 minutes. If others are still awake, let your family know that this is *your* downtime and not to interrupt you unless there's an emergency.

- **Use tools during high-stress days.** We've all had those evenings when the mind spins too much to sleep. It helps to have some effective strategies in place when this happens. These can include deep breathing for 5 to 8 cycles or listening to a brief guided meditation. These tools are surprisingly effective at activating the parasympathetic system, which halts the clenched stomach and sweaty palms of the fight-or-flight response. Another technique that helps me is the nurturing moment, a skill I learned from the Emory University Cognitively-Based Compassion Training course. This involves remembering a moment in your life where you felt at peace, loved, or taken care of and then visualizing that moment. Think about it deeply, noting who was there, what you saw, and even what you heard or smelled. For me, this moment took place at a home in the mountains that my sister and I once rented for a couple of days. The view of the mountains, the clouds, and even the sounds of birds chirping helped me feel calmer and more grounded.

- **Write it out.** Writing helps me in those late-night moments when The List appears in my mind. I know from experience that writing things down can help decrease my anxiety that I might forget these things by morning. Writing gives you a way to download the information and ideas in a place other than your mind so you can rest.

Caffeine Intake

It's also important to be strategic about your intake of caffeine during the day. It's best to stop caffeine consumption by noon. Drinking beverages with caffeine past that time may alter your sleep later on that evening. Although this can vary from person to person, know what time is best for you to stop consuming caffeinated beverages. Caffeine can be found in surprising places, including green tea and diet drinks. For some people, even the caffeine in dark chocolate can interfere with sleep.

Alcohol Consumption

In the case of alcohol, many people believe they sleep better when they've had a drink or 2, but alcohol causes sedation, which is a different state than sleep and interferes with the many important functions the brain performs at night. Alcohol also activates the fight-or-flight response, waking you up frequently during the night and interfering with rapid eye movement sleep, or dream sleep, which scientists believe plays an important role in emotional and mental health.

A SCREEN BREAK

Monika had trouble sleeping at night and started every workday feeling anxious and overwhelmed. She made a decision to stop checking her phone after 9:00 pm and to wait until 8:00 am to check it again. This allowed her to shower, wake her kids, and feed them breakfast first. She worried that her colleagues would complain that she wasn't accessible enough. But to her surprise, no one seemed to notice. The new routine improved her sleep at night because she wasn't fretting about the emails she'd read right before bed, and it allowed her to be more peaceful and present for her kids in the morning.

Some sleep interruption is inevitable, such as when your children are sick, or an elderly parent is in the hospital. But it's smart to minimize any disruptions within your control. Send pets to another room to sleep, for example, so their movements and noises don't wake you. If you or your spouse snores, talk to your doctor about a sleep study to check for the possibility of sleep apnea, a cause of chronic, severe sleep deprivation. Putting in the effort to establish sleep as a priority can yield big benefits across your life.

Food

We know the importance of a balanced diet that includes a variety of vegetables and fruit, lean protein, and whole grains. There's no shortage of good information available on healthy eating. The real trick is finding quick ways to make healthy choices so you're not tempted to use the fast-food drive-through often. One friend I know washes a big box of salad greens and chops veggies such as cucumbers, red peppers, tomatoes, and onions on Sundays. He stores those ingredients in separate containers in the fridge and then can quickly assemble big salads for lunch each day, combining the veggies and topping them with canned chickpeas, beans, or a little bit of canned tuna for protein. He drizzles on a light dressing and has a healthy, filling lunch daily. I'm a big fan of washing and chopping vegetables for the week on Sundays to reduce the burden of meal preparation during the week.

I often cook a big batch of chili or lentil soup on Sunday and prepare another meal such as a casserole to put in the fridge. My family eats the soup or chili on Sunday with a salad and bread, the casserole on Monday, and leftovers on Tuesday. On Wednesdays we throw together a quick meal such as pasta or a stir fry, and I usually do something easy like tacos on Thursday. That gets us to Friday, our take-out night. Saturdays may be upside down, such as breakfast for dinner (eggs and waffles and smoothie), since we typically have activities most of the day, or sometimes the kids might choose the meal. It could be mac 'n' cheese, as long as there is a veggie (such as boiled broccoli or green beans) and a protein to make it complete. This little bit of planning makes mealtimes easier and moves us smoothly through most weeks. Keeping your fridge and pantry stocked with healthy snacks that you can grab easily, such as chickpea hummus and baby carrots; mixed nuts; yogurt; hard-boiled eggs; and fruit such as apples, grapes, and berries, also helps you make healthier choices when you're rushed and hungry.

Water

It comes as no surprise to anyone that water is the recommended drink of choice on a daily basis. Drinking plenty of water has been shown to reduce the risk of recurrent urinary tract infections in women, and 1 study that looked at the results of more than 33 existing studies on dehydration found that even mild dehydration can affect focus and energy. Staying hydrated is a simple way to stay sharp and energized. The standard recommendation is 8 glasses a day. There are phone apps and fun water bottles that can help you track how much you sip daily. I recommend carrying a large water bottle around to remind you to drink. If you work at a computer, keep a large glass of water next to you at your desk and replenish it frequently. Always have a large glass of water at your bedside. One tip that works for me is to drink 2 glasses of water each morning before I have my coffee. This way I start the day ahead of the game. Another simple guideline is to drink enough water that your urine is light yellow. Dark yellow urine (similar to the color of a school bus) may be a sign you're not consuming enough water.

Physical Activity

When it pertains to your physical health, it's not necessary to be a marathoner or triathlete—although big goals can be motivating. But it is well known that adults should aim for about 30 minutes of physical activity a day, 5 or more times a week. And it doesn't have to involve a gym membership or treadmill; you can simply log 30 minutes of brisk walking each day, or break your movement into 3 chunks of 10 minutes each throughout the day. Find online workout videos that you enjoy—yoga or barre workouts or dancing. Another possibility is smartphone fitness apps; a few apps offer an intense full-body workout in just 7 minutes a day using only your body weight and no equipment.

As you're considering your physical activity options, think about forms of movement that have been especially fun at different moments in your life. Are there ways you can recapture that fun as an adult? Exercise doesn't have to be grim. Consider grabbing a buddy to work out with. A group of my friends decided to "run the year" in 2019, essentially working together to log 2,019 miles before the end of the year. They didn't live in the same city but kept track of each other's mileage on a running app and cheered for each other as the miles added up and they moved closer to reaching their goal. The practice motivated them and cemented their friendship.

I've learned that on the days when I'm working from home, it helps to put on workout clothes as soon as I get up in the morning. This means 1 less hurdle to cross before I exercise. On Sundays, I plan ahead and schedule my exercise on the calendar—between work meetings and my family activities. Viewing your workout in smaller time frames can also feel more manageable. I find that planning even 2 or 3 increments of 30 minutes of exercise during the week means I'm more likely to do it. If you become sidetracked with exercise or any of the fundamental habits, as we all do on occasion, be kind to yourself. Simply do your best and let the rest go.

Battling the Serenity Stealers

In my own life and in the lives of friends and the parents I meet through my pediatrics practice, there are some common habits, such as the following, that make life more complicated and stressful:

Negative Self-talk

My sense is that this is a big one for parents, moms in particular. Many of us have a personal story of a mistake we made at work, a fender bender we had on the road, a friend's birthday that we missed, or a permission slip for a child's field trip that we forgot to sign. In the face of these mistakes, we often berate ourselves for being thoughtless, forgetful, unfocused, or 1 of a hundred other negative words. We're downright mean to ourselves. It's interesting that we have zero tolerance for bullying in our schools and communities, yet many parents regularly bully themselves, speaking to themselves in a tone they would never use to talk with a sibling or close friend. It's no surprise that 1 large study found that people who engage in self-blame tend to be more at risk for mental health issues.

It's unrealistic to expect perfection from ourselves. It is vital that we adopt a new, more compassionate tone when we speak to ourselves and that we cut ourselves slack. We could blame ourselves for being late to a birthday party, but was there traffic that you didn't expect? Did your boss call you into a project that day? Or did your sister call with a crisis that you needed to help her with? All of these factors are out of our control. In fact, *most* factors are out of our control. To take full blame for something that went wrong is simply not OK. We must realize this so that we can be compassionate to ourselves, dust ourselves off, and get back on track again. Self-blame and guilt only get in our way and make us feel bad about ourselves for no reason.

Screens and Social Media

As parents, we're used to worrying about the effect of screen time on our children's health, but it's worth considering how our own use of screen time affects us as adults. A 2018 Nielsen report found that adults spent more than 11 hours a day interacting with media. Much of that media involved digital devices, though the survey included radio and podcast listening as well. In a 2020 Pew Research Center survey, 6 of 10 parents said they spend too much time on their smartphone. Moms and college-educated parents seemed to be most likely to believe this.

Another study found a significant association between screen use and moderate or severe levels of depression. Who hasn't felt a pang of envy when scrolling past photos of another family's beautiful island vacation, or a video of someone else's child's flawless piano recital? Although many of us find it fun to scroll through social media, especially at the end of the day, it's rarely an activity that truly makes us feel refreshed, stronger, or more at peace.

We all know that social media can feel addictive. It's hard to resist that little jolt of fun or drama in moments when we're tired or bored. Think of other activities that will give you a little boost, such as a lunchtime walk, listening to a favorite song, or running to the grocery store during a break. I recommend turning off the notifications on your social media apps, and, personally, at times, I've deleted the app entirely to give myself a break. And just as we work to move our children's phones out of their bedrooms, it's wise to move our own phones away from the bedside. Scrolling on social media is inviting at the end of a long day, but it can disrupt sleep. Consider moving your phone to another table in your bedroom. This makes you less likely to check social media before your feet even hit the floor.

Some people have had success engaging in social media fasts for a week or more. An organization called the *Campaign for a Commercial-Free Childhood* holds Screen-Free Week annually, encouraging families to sign off most screens for 1 week each May. Of course, homework will need to be done, including other necessary tasks for parents, that involve a computer or tablet, but the intent of the campaign is to reduce the increased daily use of streaming shows, TV channels, social media, and video games. Some families choose to unplug 1 day a week for Screen-Free Sundays, giving everyone the chance to interact without digital devices except those that are completely necessary. If that feels too difficult, you might start with just half a day, with the goal of increasing the screen-free time a little each week.

Alcohol

Kicking back with your choice of an alcoholic beverage with friends is a common way for parents to decompress. But it's important to mention the risks of using alcohol to cope with stress. As mentioned earlier, alcohol is a sedative, and drinking at night can make sleep less restorative. The Centers for Disease Control and Prevention recommends no more than 1 alcoholic drink per day for women to minimize health risks, including disrupted sleep and dehydration, as well as an increased likelihood for substance use disorder, blood pressure issues, and even breast cancer. Men are also advised by the Centers for Disease Control and Prevention to limit drinks to 2 or fewer per day. Drinking can lead to a variety of health risks, as previously stated, as well as to a higher risk for motor vehicle accidents.

A group of friends started sampling different brands of alcohol-free mocktails made with fruit and herbs to find their favorites. One of them told me that she started a ritual of pouring her favorite seltzer in a glass with ice and a lemon garnish at 5:00 pm. It became a pleasurable way to mark the end of the day without the alcohol buzz and left her with more energy to make dinner and supervise homework. In the evening, you might swap out your glass of wine for a small piece of dark chocolate. A mug of herbal tea with honey can be wonderful, especially in the winter. I have a favorite sparkling juice drink that I keep in the house for times when I want a treat, as long as my kids don't get to it first!

Anxiety

When life gets hectic and the pressure builds, sometimes anxiety can cause symptoms such as shortness of breath, a pounding heart, and feelings of panic and doom. An anxiety disorder is the most common mental health disorder in the United States, and women are almost twice as likely to develop them as men. It's important to learn how to pause in high-tension moments and to breathe deeply to ease the stress hormones that flood the body when we're stressed. Breathing and habits such as taking a walk or a jog can help counter anxiety, and cognitive behavioral therapy is also a proven tool to address and help manage it. Research shows that vitamin D (such as from sunlight!) can affect our moods and our circadian rhythms in positive ways by having a calming effect and reducing stress.

How we manage the negative stress in our lives can play a role in our anxiety. Buddhist teachers often use the story of the second arrow to illustrate this concept. Being hit by 1 arrow really hurts, they explain. The second arrow is the story we tell ourselves about that first arrow, and we have at least some control over how much pain it causes. Will we rehash the painful experience over and over or berate ourselves or others, making the pain worse? Or will we try not to dwell so painfully on what happened, learn strategies to manage the pain and cope, and eventually move forward? I think about my sister who backed out of her driveway one afternoon to take her son to a music lesson. Suddenly she heard a loud crunching sound. Imagine how shocked she was when she discovered that she had run over her son's guitar, which she'd forgotten to load into the trunk for his lesson. She was so angry with herself. She berated herself for days, and that story or rehashing became the painful second arrow. Mistakes happen, but when we have a little compassion for ourselves, we are better able to move forward and ensure the next time we handle situations differently.

Understanding that there will always be things out of our control can really help relieve some of the anxiety and even guilt in some situations. In my sister's case, chances are that there were many factors that led to her distraction. Also, remember that life is not perfect, and no one has a perfect life, no matter what people share or how their social media accounts look. It's completely normal to experience bad days or to make mistakes.

Using the Basic Pillars

The basic pillars can help ground us and make us better able to deal with the stress that life sends our way. These pillars were built into society via traditions over hundreds of years, but with our fast-paced lives, they have become less and less a priority. By pulling these back in, we can use these aspects to help us cope and be whole.

Community

Who is your squad? Who are the people you can count on to share your joys and lend a hand in a challenging time? This is worth reflecting on; a lot of research shows that social support is an important buffer in stressful times, yet many people lack that kind of network. If that's true for you, what can you do to build community around you? It rarely happens overnight, but community building is worthwhile. Who in your neighborhood or at work seems like a kindred spirit? Who do you want to know better? Anne's story shows that these connections can be a lifeline. She joined a group of neighbors who met at 6:00 am twice a week to jog around the neighborhood. When

Anne's 12-year-old son had a serious bike accident and spent a week in the hospital, the jogging group mobilized, helping drive her younger children to school and providing meals. Their kindness made a difficult time easier for Anne and her family and brought the group members closer.

Kindness

When we focus our attention on helping others, it not only takes our mind off our own worries, it reminds us that we're not the only ones with challenges. It also helps us connect with others more deeply. We move beyond everyday small talk and step into the lives of others in a meaningful way. It's a matter of picking up groceries for an elderly neighbor when you're at the store. It's posting an inspirational quote on your social media account or checking on a friend who is going through a divorce. It all counts. And it has physical and mental health benefits, too.

Kindness can also shift the way we look at things. When we see others who may not have what we have, it makes us realize and appreciate what we do have instead of focusing on what we don't. When my dad had brain surgery and my teenage son was suddenly hospitalized with a serious illness, I was in a very stressed space. But then I heard about my friend who had cancer and took her a meal. While acknowledging my own emotions and not minimizing what I was going through, I found that helping someone else allowed me an attitude shift, prompting me to think about the many things I'm grateful for.

Saying No

Many parents can admit that they always commit and say yes to any opportunity that arises. When asked to help with baking cupcakes or soliciting donations for a fundraiser, or leading teacher appreciation efforts at school, or taking on an extra project at work, we rarely say no. Our time quickly gets eaten up, and we're left frosting cupcakes in the kitchen at 2:00 am instead of getting the sleep we need. It's important to acknowledge this yes tendency—and to make a habit of pausing to decide what really deserves our time. A friend of mine was always the go-to guy for help with stuff around the house, and he was often pulled into helping others, such as helping a friend move, fixing someone's lawn mower, or coaching the local kid's soccer team. One day he realized that having a full-time job and consistently assisting with other tasks took a lot of time away from him being able to unwind. And that time was so necessary to replenish himself and to be the best dad he strove to be.

I also remember the example of Lindsay, who'd been asked by her children's school to run the annual fundraising dinner for the third year in a row. Lindsay had managed it well in the past, but this year she wanted the time and energy for personal projects. Lindsay told the principal, "I'm sorry, but I'm not able to run the dinner again." It was difficult for her to resist the urge to offer a dozen awkward excuses or big apologies, but she simply let her statement stand. Since then, she's grown stronger in her ability to say no. Saying no allows her to spend more time on the activities that matter the most to her. For those of us who always feel bad about saying no, look for alternatives. Are you able to take on another smaller task instead so you feel as if you are still doing your part? Can you recommend someone else to bake the classroom cupcakes, someone who is trying to make connections, allowing them to meet new people at school?

Slowing Down

In a busy life, it's often our instinct to rush through our tasks. Some days it feels as if it is the only way to accomplish even half the items on the must-do list. But slowing down some elements of your day may help you—and your children—cope better on stressful days. Michelle, a busy working mom of 4, decided to make slowing down her new practice for 1 year. The biggest change she made was committing to no longer rushing while driving, which was not only safer but also made her feel less anxious and judgmental of other drivers. She also tried to slow down her conversations with others, which she found led to feeling more connected to her children, her coworkers, and her spouse. Looking back, she says that slowing down did not delay her but allowed her a little more space to breathe.

How to Fill Your Cup

One of the keys of self-care is adopting habits that restore and recharge you, or fill your cup, as the saying goes. I suggest you write down a list of activities that you find grounding and refreshing. Ideally, some of these activities can be completed in just 5 to 10 minutes, allowing you to take restorative mini breaks during your craziest of days. These might include listening to a few minutes of a podcast or funny audiobook (autobiographies of comics are great picks) while completing chores such as the dishes or laundry. Consider mini doses of nature, such as 10 minutes of gardening outside or tending to a houseplant. Perform quick acts of kindness, such as buying a stranger's coffee when you pay for your own or making a $10 donation to a charity you admire. Leave a fresh drawing pad open on your desk or the kitchen counter next to a pack of markers; pause occasionally to doodle. Check out a book of poetry from the library and read a poem a day. If you enjoy sudoku or crosswords, aim to complete 1 over the course of the day, working at it just a minute or a 2 at a time. What would be on your fill-my-cup list?

I enjoy scheduling social dates during the week, such as phone chats with friends or family or meeting them for hikes. You deserve connection time, and it must be a priority. I do this every Sunday morning. It makes me happier and a better mom to my kids. Scheduling these in advance makes me feel less overwhelmed about feeling disconnected and helps to plan each day of the week. It also gives me other things to look forward to, and I am comforted knowing I will be my best calm self when those times arrive.

You Are Not Alone

If you only take away 2 ideas from this chapter, I hope it's these. First, you are not alone in feeling stressed and overwhelmed; no matter how picture-perfect others' lives may look on the outside, we are all struggling in some ways with life. Second, taking care of yourself is not a luxury. It's a nonnegotiable necessity of parenting. We all want more from life than a to-do list and deadlines and hours spent juggling the schedule of practices and tutoring sessions and music lessons. Your self-care is not only key to helping your child thrive but it's also how you claim the healthier, more meaningful life that you deserve as well.

Toolbox Takeaways for Replenishing Your Cup

TAKEAWAY 1: **Support**

Call or text a friend who understands the challenges of parenting and can provide a listening ear when you need it.

TAKEAWAY 2: **Relax**

Find easy ways to relax such as reading or listening to music, audiobooks, or podcasts while sitting under a favorite tree.

Change up your daily routes when walking your dog or take a walk around the block. I love to do spin and yoga and will even take my yoga mat outside when it's nice.

TAKEAWAY 3: **Laugh**

Laughter is an automatic stress buster, and short, funny online videos are also an easy way to bond with teens and tweens. One of my patients and his mom maintain a playlist of their favorite funny videos, including some fantastic clips of laughing foxes in a fox sanctuary.

TAKEAWAY 4: **Meditate**

It's no surprise that meditation can make you less reactive and help you focus. Downloading guided meditation apps dedicated to decreasing anxiety is a great way to start the habit, providing a voice to guide you through the meditation. Many guided meditations take just minutes to complete.

TAKEAWAY 5: **Read**

Choosing a book over your social media feed is almost always the healthier choice. Keep a novel in your bag to reach for in the moments when you're tempted to scroll. If you can read only a few pages at a time, don't sweat it. Consider gathering to discuss the book with friends when you're done.

QUIZ

Does Your Family Have a Plan in Place for Crises?

1. What is your honest view of your family's mental well-being?
   - a. My family is basically fine. I don't see us encountering mental health problems. (5 points)
   - b. Everyone struggles at some point in life. We're fine right now, but I can reach out to a mental health professional if someone in my family is dealing with an issue. (3 points)
   - c. We don't need to reach crisis levels to address mental wellness at our house. We discuss mental health topics regularly and prefer to consider potential trouble spots before they become full-blown problems. (0 points)

2. Does your family have an established relationship with at least 1 mental health professional such as a psychologist or counselor or a primary care doctor who can help with mental health?

    a. Yes (0 points)

    b. No, but I know who to call to connect us with a mental health professional. (2 points)

    c. No (5 points)

3. When was the last time you and your child communicated about what either of you was thinking or feeling?

    a. Today (0 points)

    b. Sometime in the last 2 or 3 days (1 point)

    c. Sometime in the last week (2 points)

    d. Sometime in the last month (3 points)

    e. A few times a year (4 points)

    f. Never (5 points)

4. In an emergency, do you have nearby friends or family you could call for help?

    a. No. We're basically on our own. (5 points)

    b. Yes. I believe we could rely on at least 1 friend or family member who could help in a time of crisis. (3 points)

    c. Yes. We have a network of people who would help us in a time of trouble. (0 points)

5. Have you and your child discussed difficult topics such as suicide, substance use disorder, depression, or sexual abuse?

    a. Yes. We talk about these topics regularly. (0 points)

    b. Yes, although it's been a while. We probably need to revisit these topics again. (1 point)

    c. No, but I'm willing to talk about them if I have tips on constructive ways to discuss these issues. (4 points)

    d. No, but I know these topics are covered at school. (5 points)

Add up your score. Total _____

What Your Score Means

0 to 8 points: It sounds like your family has useful, beneficial habits and structures in place to help you face the ups and downs of life, including the mental health crisis of a child. It's important to do what you can to keep lines of communication open and to make moods and feelings a regular topic of conversation. Make it clear to your kid that they can come to you anytime they are having trouble coping and that you will do everything you can to help.

9 to 16 points: You know how to find help for your child in an emergency, but it's important to make mental health a regular topic of conversation in your home. Let kids know that there's no shame in feeling low or anxious, that it's important for them to speak up if they need help, and that you're there to help if they're having trouble. In this chapter, we cover some common mental health crises and ways you can help your child if they're struggling.

17 to 25 points: The fact is that many families will face some kind of mental health crisis sooner or later. Unfortunately, no family is immune to anxiety, depression, or other mood disorders. In this chapter, we cover information on the types of crises kids and parents sometimes face. The point is not to add to your own anxiety but to raise your awareness and give you effective strategies to cope if a crisis emerges. Let's get started.

CHAPTER 8

Your Child's Mental Health: What to Do During a Crisis

've talked about the mental emotional toolbox that our children and teens need to help them reduce stress in daily life. But what happens when things become *really* difficult, and your child experiences a significant crisis? Events that may feel especially troubling to parents are learning that your child has an eating disorder or substance use disorder or that they are depressed or having suicidal thoughts. When it's evident that your kid is truly distressed, what are the best ways to care for them and help them cope and heal, while also holding yourself together?

Life is tough. Sometimes, despite parents' best efforts, families can be blindsided and experience unexpected changes. As a pediatrician, I've walked with many families through difficult, unexpected circumstances. And if I can share 1 insight from those experiences, it's this truth: The situations that rock our world can truly happen to *any* of us.

Lucy's Story

A parent called me 1 day about his 14-year-old daughter Lucy. During a school meeting, the principal had explained that Lucy and her friend had been caught vaping in the girls' bathroom. When confronted by her parents, Lucy started sobbing uncontrollably and admitted to cutting herself and having thoughts of suicide.

(continued)

Depressed mood and substance use are often inter-twined and often come together. Suicidal thoughts and sui-cide attempts are not as isolated as we may think. In fact, the Centers for Disease Control and Prevention reports that the rate of suicide among people aged 10 to 24 years increased significantly between 2007 and 2018. The factors leading to thoughts of suicide are varied and can occur even in the most well-put-together families that appear perfect on social media. It can happen to any of us.

To find out more about the mental health crises that families can face, I turned to 2 mental health professionals who I respect tremendously: psychologist Linda Pak Bruner, PhD, who has a private practice in Atlanta, Georgia, and child psychiatrist Smitha Bhandari, MD, who sees patients through the Path Group of Atlanta LLC. Both have helped hundreds of families navigate mental health challenges, and I've drawn on their experienced perspectives as they describe some of the signs that suggest a child or teen is struggling. They also suggest steps parents can take if they see evidence of trouble.

My intent with this chapter is not to worry you unneces-sarily. Instead, my hope is to provide you with a set of resources that can be a source of strength if you ever need them. Even if your family life is currently peaceful, you can refer back to this information later if significant challenges arise.

Suicidal Thoughts or Suicide Attempts

Teens are known for their impulsivity; the brain is one of the last organs to develop, and teens are less able to access areas of the brain responsible for insight and self-regulation. As a result, teens are more likely than adults to make split-second decisions that put their lives at risk. This doesn't mean that they can't make decisions that are rational. It just means that, because of incomplete connections, emotions can override the logical part of the brain when they are stressed. For example, they might suddenly harm themselves in response to mean comments on social media or an embarrassing experience at school, Bhandari explains.

Rates of suicide among young people aged 10 to 24 have risen alarmingly—by nearly 60% between 2007 and 2018. Researchers also saw an increase in suicidal thinking and suicide attempts among adolescents during the COVID-19 pandemic, as communities went into lockdown. Studies show that the majority of teens who died by suicide met the criteria for a mood disorder such as anxiety or depression. If you notice signs of anxiety or depression in your kid, it's important to help them get treatment and help them manage the disorder.

Signs to Watch For

- Your child/teen has strong reactions to relationship difficulties or becomes particularly upset in response to certain friend interactions.
- Your child/teen suddenly seems withdrawn.
- You see your child's mood shift after they spend time on social media platforms.
- Your child/teen has lost interest in activities that they used to enjoy.
- Your child/teen talks about death or suicide.
- Your child/teen has a sudden, unexpected decline in grades.
- Your child/teen says they have a friend who is having suicidal thoughts.
- Your child/teen initiates alcohol or substance use.

Taking Action Now

- **Act quickly.** If your child tells you they are considering suicide, or they make a suicidal gesture, take them seriously; do not dismiss this as teen melodrama. Call your pediatrician or a mental health professional *immediately*. If you don't currently have a relationship with a pediatrician or mental health professional and you're worried that your child could hurt themselves, consider taking them to a local emergency department for help.
- **Remove guns from the equation.** According to the American Academy of Pediatrics, the safest home is one without guns. Research shows that teens who live in homes with guns are more likely to harm themselves than teens in homes without them are. Remove any guns from the house or ensure that they are stored away safely, locked and unloaded with the ammunition stored separately. Medications and alcohol should also be locked away where your kid can't access them.
- **Remove substances from the home.** Substances such as alcohol or cannabis can have mind-altering effects on mood.
- **Try to talk.** Make an effort to engage your child and find out specifics about how they're feeling and what they're thinking. If your kid doesn't want to talk with you—a common dynamic for many teens and parents—enlist the help of another adult you and your child both trust, such as an aunt or uncle.

Preventive Measures to Take Now

Discuss Mood With Your Kids

I recommend that you talk to your kids early about mood disorders such as anxiety and depression, as well as suicide. With my own children, I've brought up suicide during our regular discussions including bullying, harassment, or inappropriate touching. Make sure your child knows that if they hear a friend talking about wanting to harm themselves, they should tell you or another trusted adult immediately. And make sure that you have a relationship with a mental health specialist before any issues arise so that you can reach out to them as needed.

Watch for Signs of Bullying

Being bullied in person or online can negatively affect a child's physical and emotional well-being. If your child suddenly stops wanting to go to school or has an abrupt decline in school performance, ask questions. Other signs of bullying include lost or destroyed clothing or other belongings and the sudden disappearance of friends.

Pay Extra Attention After a Friend's Death

Sometimes suicide can appear contagious among teens. This doesn't mean you shouldn't talk about it. Have an open dialogue about how your child is feeling about the suicide. Point out that the child or teen who died probably didn't know how much they were loved or that they didn't realize that there is always help available.

Encourage Movement

Physical activity is one of the most effective remedies for depression, so encourage your kids to find ways to work out 30 minutes at a time most days of the week. Taking a walk or bike ride alone or with family and friends can help lift their mood.

Key for Parents: If your child is suicidal and requires treatment, it is important to get support for yourself. A great resource is the National Suicide Prevention Lifeline (https://suicidepreventionlifeline.org). Also, lean on your inner circle to see if they can help with tasks such as meal preparation or rides for your other children. Do not be afraid to ask for help.

A COMMUNITY COPES WITH LOSS

Several years ago, multiple teenage boys died by suicide just a few weeks apart in a community near me. Parents and teachers were stunned—and alarmed that vulnerable teens seemed to be copying one another. These deaths led many parents to worry about their own teenage boys. What were they thinking and feeling? Was it possible that they, too, were quietly suffering from depression or anxiety and not reaching out for help? Dr Pak Bruner indicated that some parents contacted her to set up appointments for their children. They hoped that as a psychologist and therapist she could determine if there were any signs of mood disorders that they as parents might be missing.

Even if a child is not experiencing a crisis, most can benefit from the sounding board of a smart, attentive mental health professional who has the skill set to help those who are struggling to manage their emotional state. Establishing a good relationship with a therapist can be helpful in the event that your child needs help down the road. If you are hesitant to seek therapy because of the cost, look for mental health professionals who offer sliding scale fees. Some insurance plans cover a set number of mental health visits each year; call your insurer to ask for a list of the practitioners who are in network.

Self-harm (Cutting)

Self-harm is a disturbing set of behaviors in which kids or teens intentionally cut or carve their skin with sharp objects or scratch or bruise themselves as a way to cope with or distract themselves from intense emotional pain. Children and teens may self-harm in response to experiences such as rejection, a breakup, or bullying. "Some people say that the physical pain of cutting distracts from emotional pain, or is in some way easier to experience, feel, and recover from than emotional pain," explained Dr Bhandari. Other times a child will hurt their body as a way to punish themselves for perceived faults.

Most children who self-harm are not trying to kill themselves. But cuts or scars on your child's arm can be signs of a suicide attempt. If you see evidence of cuts or scars, Dr Bhandari recommends connecting your child with a mental health professional to determine what's going on.

Signs to Watch For

- Your child has unexplained cuts, scratches, bruises, or burns.
- Your child wears long sleeves or pants, even in hot weather, and doesn't want to be seen in a swimsuit or other revealing clothing.
- Your child experiences a significant change in mood or behavior.
- Your child possesses multiple razors or other sharp objects that can be used for self-harm.
- Your child creates art, stories, or poems that glorify death, blood, wounds, or sharp objects.
- Your child spends long periods of time alone in their room or in the bathroom, more than typical for your child.

Taking Action Now

1. **Call your pediatrician or mental health professional.** If you see evidence that your kid is engaging in self-harm, contact your pediatrician for a referral or a psychotherapist. These experts can offer guidance about next steps.
2. **Don't ignore evidence of self-harm.** This is a sign that your child is experiencing significant emotional

distress. Act as soon as you can to help your child. Don't look away.

3. **Talk to your child.** Sometimes it is not easy to bring up a tough topic. But I believe that being direct (and as calm as possible) is the best policy. Let your child know that you are very concerned and will work with them to get help. Again, try not to be angry or accusatory, and work to gain their trust. Listen closely to what they say, even if you are scared or angry about their behavior.

4. **Bring up the topic multiple times.** Your child may deny that there's a problem, become angry or defensive, or shut down. Don't give up. If you suspect that your teen is hurting themselves, remove them from any harmful situation, stay with them, and bring up the topic again. You may ask another family member or trusted coach or teacher to speak to them if you feel like you aren't able to get through to your kid.

Preventive Measures to Take Now

Let Your Child Know You Are Always There for Them

This bears repeating: I believe strongly that it's important to let your kid know that you are there whenever they need you. Also, let them know that they can come to you for help if a friend ever reveals that they are hurting themselves.

Talk About Healthy Ways to Cope

Discuss healthy ways to handle difficult feelings or tough times. Make a list of ways to relieve the pressure of painful feelings, such as going for a run, shooting baskets, calling a friend, or watching a funny movie to lift their spirits.

Check In on Hard Days

When your child is undergoing an experience that might be painful—such as a breakup or an unsatisfactory score on a test—don't let them spend hours alone in their room. Check in regularly, saying that you know they might be experiencing difficult feelings. Ask if they'd like to chat or go for a walk.

Key for Parents: Self-harm and cutting are shocking and scary for parents. Learn what you can about these behaviors so you can be equipped to help your kid. I also like this advice from my colleague, Dr Bhandari: "It's also OK to say to your child, 'I don't know how to handle this. Let's figure out who can help us and see if they can help us understand what's going on.' It's OK to reach out for help."

Eating Disorders

Eating disorders are problematic behaviors around food and eating. They can take multiple forms, but common forms include anorexia (restricting eating on purpose), bulimia (binge eating, followed by forcing the body to throw up, using laxatives, or exercising excessively to make up for the overeating), and binge eating disorder (eating rapidly, without hunger, to the point of extreme fullness, at least once a week for 3 months). Eating disorders affect both boys and girls, often go hand in hand with other mental health disorders such as anxiety and depression, and can be life-threatening. Kids who are lesbian, gay, bisexual, transgender, queer or questioning, asexual or allied, or intersex (LGBTQIA+) are often at higher risk for eating disorders. People with eating disorders can have all types of body shapes and weights. If your child does not follow their growth chart as expected, talk to your pediatrician about the possibility of an eating disorder.

Signs to Watch For

- Your child/teen suddenly loses weight or doesn't follow their growth chart.
- Your child/teen changes their diet. Sometimes this may take the form of choosing to eat vegetarian, vegan, or gluten-free diets.
- Your child/teen makes frequent bathroom visits during or after meals.
- Your child/teen participates in sports that emphasize weight, such as dancing, wrestling, track, or gymnastics.
- Your child/teen no longer wants to eat with the family.
- Your child/teen dramatically changes their exercise routine.
- Your child/teen wears many layers of clothing even when its warm outside.
- Your daughter's period becomes irregular or stops.

Taking Action Now

1. **Find help immediately.** Ask your pediatrician to refer you to a mental health professional with expertise in treating eating disorders. Don't be tempted to let this go; your child has a better chance of full recovery the sooner an eating disorder is diagnosed and treated.

2. **Keep talking.** As with the other crises included in this chapter, it's important to maintain open communication with your child and to respond as calmly and openly as you can to the possibility that they have an eating disorder. Let your kid know that you are committed to working together to find them help.

3. **Arrange for a medical checkup.** Some families believe their work is done once they've connected their child with a mental health professional. Ensure that your child is also seen by their pediatrician and that they

receive a full checkup to determine if they have any
physical consequences of their disordered eating.

Preventive Measures to Take Now

Promote Healthy Body Image

Praise your child's healthy, strong body, and talk about the
variety of body shapes and sizes. Discuss harmful messages
in the media about weight and body types and point out
friends, family members, and celebrities with healthy attitudes about nutrition and weight.

Promote Healthy Eating

Discuss how what you eat influences how you feel. Encourage your child to eat when hungry. Have dinner together as
a family as often as you can, since this is a place where kids
can develop healthy attitudes about food.

Key for Parents: Please know that parents do not cause
eating disorders in their child but rather are essential in
helping their child heal.

Bullying

Bullying is now understood to be so much more than a
group of kids teasing or being mean to another kid. The bullied child can be deeply affected emotionally, physically, and
academically. The definition of bullying is when 1 or more
kids repeatedly harass a child who is seen as less powerful,
perhaps because they dress differently, learn differently, are
of a different color or race, or have gender differences. The
intimidation can include physical harassment in the form of
hitting or tripping or verbal abuse such as name-calling or
comments that are sexual in nature, or it can involve spread-
ing rumors about a child and purposely excluding them

from social events. Bullying can take place in person or, commonly, on social media or via text message. All parties, including the victim, the child who bullies, and even the bystander can experience lasting effects.

Signs to Watch For

- Your child does not want to go to school.
- Your child seems especially upset after spending time online or on their phone.
- Your child's academic performance has declined.
- Your child has trouble sleeping, has nightmares, or complains of frequent stomachaches or headaches.
- Your child has low self-esteem.
- Your child's social circle suddenly shrinks or changes.

Taking Action Now

1. **Listen calmly.** If your child tells you they are being bullied, or you suspect that they are being harassed, ask them for details and listen as carefully and as calmly as you can. Patient listening can encourage your child to confide in you and might prompt them to share more details. Ask your child what you can do to help.
2. **Write it down.** Make notes about what your child tells you, with dates. Take screenshots of any online bullying. These can be helpful if you speak with school officials.
3. **Know your school's policy.** Educate yourself and your child. Ask to see the school's rules about bullying and read them carefully.
4. **Consider talking to school officials.** Encourage your child to talk with a school counselor or another adult at school who they trust. Empowering them to handle

this can build their confidence. If your child is too upset or not yet ready to handle this on their own, accompany them after school to discuss this problem with their teacher or other school official.

5. **Make a plan to deal with people who bully.** Brainstorm a plan with your kid. Each family will have its own strategies. My kids and I developed a 3-step plan: If someone bullies you, first politely ask them to walk away. The second time, speak more assertively and ask them to walk away again. The third time call in a teacher or other adult to resolve the situation. Of course, I tell my kids that if there is any worry that a person who bullies will physically harm them, they should go directly to step 3 and approach an adult.

Preventive Measures to Take Now

Encourage Kindness

From an early age, teach your child the importance of showing respect for and kindness to others. Continue to remind your child as they grow older that this is an important value in your family.

Value Self-respect

Just as you would encourage your child to respect others, encourage self-respect, too. I talk often with my own kids about the importance of walking with confidence and not allowing people to bully you or others.

Talk About the Role of the Bystander

Discuss with your child how they might safely intervene if another child is being bullied: Can they speak up or alert an adult such as a teacher, school counselor, or principal?

Monitor Your Child's Social Media Accounts

I recommend that parents establish a presence on social media platforms so they can follow their child's accounts and monitor interactions with their peers.

Key for Parents: Hearing that your child is being bullied can be very upsetting to parents and may trigger memories of your own experiences of being bullied (or bullying others). Before you react, listen carefully to your child and find out what they need most from you.

Substance Use Disorder

Kids may encounter drugs, alcohol, or cigarettes in middle school or high school. Unfortunately, some kids may even encounter them in elementary school. During these periods, children and teens want more than anything to fit in with their peers, which can increase their chances of making unhealthy decisions such as experimenting with drugs or drinking to excess. It may take kids only 1 or 2 times of "experimenting" before a drug or alcohol becomes purposeful and is no longer experimentation. Prescription drug misuse is one of the most common forms of substance misuse among teens, so I advise parents to keep medications such as painkillers and anti-anxiety medications locked up and out of reach. Research has shown that the earlier a child or teen tries a substance, the more likely going back to the substance will be intentional. A substance use disorder is much more likely to begin at age 13 versus age 16 or age 25. Many states are now legalizing marijuana, which can make access to this drug easier. "Kids know a lot about what's going on in the world and about recreational and medicinal use of marijuana in different states," stated Dr Bhandari. "It can be hard for adolescents to navigate. They think, 'If other people, such as parents or siblings, are using it for medicine or recreationally, why can't I use it?'" This makes frequent conversations about drugs particularly important. Also, substance use disorder may signal that your child is experiencing severe anxiety, depression, or another mental health issue that needs addressing and treatment.

Signs to Watch For

- Your child experiences sudden changes in behavior, appearance, or eating habits or starts hanging out with a new group of friends.
- Your child appears to be under the influence of drugs or alcohol.
- Your child withdraws from family.
- Your child has difficulty getting up for school.
- Your child's grades drop.
- Your child owns drug-related tools such as pipes or lighters.

Taking Action Now

1. **Talk about any concerns.** If you suspect that your child/ teen is drinking alcohol or smoking, be direct but as calm as you can be. Give your child specific details about what you've noticed—the smell of pot smoke in your child's hair or the fact that they seemed hung over—to back up your concerns. Explain why the substance use is a problem. First and foremost, it is illegal and not a healthy outlet. Getting caught with illegal substances can affect a college application or a job application. Work to maintain your teen's trust and encourage honesty.

2. **Get medical help.** If you think your child could have a substance use disorder, contact your pediatrician for guidance; they can refer you to a mental health professional who specializes in substance use disorders.

3. **Discuss driving under the influence.** Talk about the real dangers of riding in a car driven by someone who has been drinking alcohol or smoking pot. Encourage them to call you or another adult you both trust for a ride anytime their driver is under the influence. Some families I work with have established a 24- or 48-hour amnesty period before their teen is required to share the details of what happened with their parents.

4. **Prepare now for questions.** Get ready—your child is likely to ask about your own experiences with alcohol and drugs, so consider how you'll answer. I want to stress that you don't have to share stories of your own youthful indiscretions. But if you do decide to share, offer what you learned in the process and try hard not to glamorize drinking or drug use in front of your children.

Preventive Measures to Take Now

Set Clear Rules

I recommend that you have concrete rules around drinking and drug use and that you explain why you've established these rules. For example, "I do not want you to try or drink alcohol until you are 21. Being intoxicated can make it difficult to keep yourself safe." Most kids do best when they know the limits and they have a sense of what will happen if they break the rules. Let your kids know that if they are dependent on 1 substance, such as alcohol, it makes them more likely to become dependent on another. As the parent, it is critical that your child knows that if they are ever in a situation and need help, despite having potentially broken the rules, you will be there for them.

Increase Drug Awareness

Talk with your children about what is happening with substance use disorder and how it is not difficult to get into dangerous situations. With more than 70,000 deaths per year from opioid-related use, it is key for kids to be aware of the dangers. Additionally, many pills that may be handed out at teen parties can be laced with lethal synthetic drugs including fentanyl. Advise your kids to never accept a drink or any type of drug from other people, even if they may be a friend. I advise my kids to always get their own drink and never accept any type of pill or marijuana gummy from anyone. Have these conversations frequently and answer any questions they may have.

Keep the Conversation Going

Think beyond a single conversation about alcohol and drugs. Instead, let your kid know that you want to keep talking, that you plan to bring up the topic on a regular basis, and that they are welcome to ask you questions anytime. I advise checking in if you notice significant shifts in your teen's mood or friend groups, for example.

Ask for Details

Each time your child leaves the house, ask them where they will be and with whom. Aim to meet your child's friends and consider connecting with the friend's parents, if only to get a sense of their family rules and expectations. One group of friends established a text thread when their children began hanging out together, and this became helpful in knowing their whereabouts or access to more information when one of the boys came home intoxicated.

Require Check-ins

Ask your child to find you for a chat after they arrive home at the end of a night out with friends. A face-to-face conversation gives you an opportunity to both check in on how the night went—Did they have fun? Do they enjoy these friends? Do they seem upset?—and notice if they are under the influence. Knowing that they will have to talk with you may prevent your kid from testing the limits and engaging in risky behaviors.

Note Any Family History

If you or anyone in your family has a history of substance use disorder, let your child know. Explain that their genes could put them at risk for a substance use disorder.

Key for Parents: Many parents stumble here because of their own history of drug or alcohol use, and they fear being seen as a hypocrite. Try not to let your child's questions derail you from your goal—preventing your child from drinking or using drugs before they reach adulthood and their brain development is complete.

Paul's Story

Paul always took his classes very seriously. Because he had a goal of studying engineering in college, many of his classmates started teasing him about being a highly driven "gunner" by 10th grade. At his friend's party, Paul decided just this once to loosen up, fit in, and try vaping. By the time his parents found out, 2 months later, Paul had developed a substance use disorder. And it wasn't just nicotine he had a substance use disorder with. The first few times he vaped, the liquid was laced with K2/spice, a synthetic marijuana that can be highly addictive. Paul reached out to a psychiatrist to help him quit.

According to some studies, opiate use in adolescents has decreased over the last few years from a high of approximately 4% to less than 2%. Early marijuana or alcohol use makes it more likely someone will use opiates in young adulthood. Marijuana, alcohol, and nicotine are, by far, the substances adolescents most commonly use.

Sexual Identity and Gender Identity

When a child comes out, revealing that they are LGBTQIA+, some families are shaken. Parents may have a strong, negative response, which can be devastating for their child. Dr Pak Bruner recommends trying to maintain a neutral response, if possible. If you need some private time to cry or process what your child has told you, she advises saying something such as, "Wow! That's a lot to take in. Thank you for sharing that, but I need time to think." Step away and let them know when you'll get back to them—to talk more.

Dr Pak Bruner says she has worked with many parents who reacted negatively when their child first came out to them. She's found that they often regret that initial response and have to work hard to regain their child's trust. Children who identify as LGBTQIA+ face an increased risk of depression, suicide, and substance use disorder, but a supportive family can help reduce those risks.

Signs to Watch For

- Because LGBTQIA+ kids are at increased risk of mental health problems, watch for signs that your child is struggling with anxiety, low self-esteem, or other issues and needs to talk with a psychotherapist or counselor.
- Even if you suspect that your child is LGBTQIA+, don't confront them with questions about their sexual identity; wait for them to come to you.
- Keep track of how school and peer interactions are going for your child; be alert to signs of bullying, and be ready to advocate for your child if they need support.

Taking Action Now

1. **Listen, listen, and listen some more.** Dr Pak Bruner says that it's best for parents to try to take in the information from their child without judgment, as difficult as this can be. Attentive listening is one of the best ways to keep your child's trust and stay connected to them.

2. **Let them know that you love and support them.** Even parents who have reservations about LGBTQIA+ lifestyles can reassure their child that they love them deeply and support them. "That's a really important distinction," said Dr Bhandari. "You can acknowledge how someone feels and give them support without necessarily agreeing with them."

3. **Learn more.** Educate yourself through organizations such as PFLAG, https://pflag.org; Gender Spectrum, https://www.genderspectrum.org; the Human Rights Campaign, https://www.hrc.org; and the GSA Network, https://gsanetwork.org. These resources can help you learn about LGBTQIA+ issues, including the meaning of terms used by the LGBTQIA+ community.

Preventive Measures to Take Now

Make It Clear That You Love Them Unconditionally

Dr Pak Bruner reminds parents to get to know their children as they are, instead of how they wish they were. Also, remind your child that you love them unconditionally. They need to hear it. Be ready to talk when they are ready.

Introduce Your Child to Positive Role Models

No matter how your child identifies, acknowledge gender diversity, pointing out friends, community leaders, politicians, and other gender-diverse people you know or admire.

Find Places You Can Talk

You may have strong feelings about your child's identity. Find friends, a therapist, a support group, or other places where you can process your feelings without harming your relationship with your child.

Key for Parents: No matter how you feel about your child's sexual identity, let them know that you love them and want the best for them.

Sexual Abuse and Assault

Conversations about sexual assault—which is defined as any type of unwanted sexual attention or sexual contact—are an essential part of keeping children and teens safe. The Rape, Abuse and Incest National Network (RAINN), an antisexual assault organization, reports that "1 in 9 girls and 1 in 53 boys under the age of 18 experience sexual abuse or assault at the hands of an adult." Children and teens also need to know how to keep themselves safe in situations with their peers. In most cases, victims know the people who assault them.

Electronic devices have created new opportunities for sexual content to be shared and for young people potentially to be exploited. The sexual selfie is a problem I hear about frequently, with middle schoolers and teens sending nude or nearly nude photos of themselves to friends and then being alarmed by how fast the photos are passed to people they don't even know. One of the keys to sexual safety is talking regularly with your kids about personal boundaries, including how to maintain them and respect them.

Signs to Watch For

Children who have been sexually assaulted or abused may show signs of distress that overlap with the other crises shared in this chapter.

- Your child experiences unusual weight gain or weight loss.
- Your child has bruises or other signs of being physically abused.
- Your child has a sexually transmitted infection.
- Your child shows signs of anxiety or depression.
- Your child's grades drop suddenly.
- Your child is drinking or using drugs.
- Your child is self-harming.
- Your child is suicidal.

Taking Action Now

1. **Listen to and believe your child.** If your child comes to you to say that they have been sexually assaulted, drop everything to listen. Let them know that what happened to them is not their fault. Immediately assure them that you believe them and that you will do all you can to help them. Thank your child for coming to you to share this information.

2. **Determine next steps.** Your child's physical health should be one of your first concerns. Do they need medical care? Talk to your pediatrician, who can examine your child and also connect you with resources such as a mental health professional. Another option is to call a sexual assault hotline, such as RAINN, 800/656-4673, which is available 24 hours a day, 7 days a week to provide help.

3. **Take care of yourself.** Breathe deeply; this will likely be very difficult for you as a parent. Tell your child that you are very glad they came to you and that you want to do all that you can to help them. Get a drink of water, take a walk, or do whatever you need to regroup and continue the conversation.

Preventive Measures to Take Now

Talk About Sexual Boundaries Early and Often

When your child was a toddler, you taught them the names of their body parts and explained that some parts of the body are private, as well as what the boundaries of those private parts are. As a pediatrician, I engage in this conversation during well-child visits as well. If you didn't talk about these things when your child was little, please know that it's never too late to start the conversation. I encourage you to be brave and start talking. Remind your kids that just as others may not look at or touch these areas on their bodies, they also may not look at or touch these areas on other people.

Teach the Importance of No

Help your child understand that they can always say no if they feel uncomfortable with any physical contact with another person and that it's important to honor other people's wishes if they say no to contact with us.

Use TV Shows or Movies to Spark Conversation

TV shows or movies can offer opportunities to discuss the topic of consent. How does the main character feel about a sexual encounter in the TV show or movie? Why would it be problematic for the main character to pursue sex with someone who has passed out from drinking?

Read Up on Sexting and Discuss the Risks

Sexting has exploded in popularity, but unfortunately many teens don't fully understand how these photos can lead to trouble. I've been disturbed to learn about teens whose "harmless" nude photos originally meant for a significant other end up on porn sites and teens who end up being suspended from school or charged by police for sharing these photos. Discuss such scenarios with your children and how such photos are used by others. How would they feel if photos of them or a friend were being circulated? Discuss rules and safety around using social media and digital devices and remind them always to come to you with any questions or if they see something that makes them feel uncomfortable.

Talk About Looking Out for Friends

Discuss how to keep friends safe. Talking about the risks to your child's friends may make your children more open to these topics.

Make Listening a Habit

Remind your child that you will always listen when they come to you with questions or concerns. There are certainly days that I have to remind myself to listen carefully when 1 of my kids comes to me late at night with a problem that seems small. But I know that listening to my child in those situations is one of the keys to building their trust in me and increases the likelihood that they'll come to me in the future if they face a more significant crisis.

WHEN YOUR CHILD IS IN CRISIS

Recently I met Deirdre, a married mom of 3 girls, who had just experienced a traumatic experience: Her teenage daughter Stephanie made an attempt on her life that resulted in serious injuries. When I asked Deirdre what advice she could offer to other parents of children in crisis, she offered 3 pieces of wisdom.

Family Medical Leave. This gave Deirdre the freedom to oversee her daughter's recovery process. Talk with your employer about intermittent and long-term federal and employer-sponsored medical leave policies.

Confide in Trusted Family or Friends. "You will need folks you can call anytime for help with meals or watching your other children," she explained.

Prioritize Routine and Recovery Rather Than Rules. Talk with your child and their treatment team to identify coping strategies and behaviors that will help your whole family ride the wave of your child's mental illness. It may be watching a movie together once a week or eating a meal together once a day are the only routines you can manage when times are tough. "This may not be the family life you imagined," Deirdre said. "But if your child feels safe, this promotes her recovery and family harmony, and that's enough."

You Are Not Alone in This Moment

If you are a parent who is in the midst of caring for a child in distress, I encourage you to visit Chapter 7, which covers the importance of replenishing your own cup so that you have the energy and resourcefulness to advocate for your child.

In my own times of distress, I often reflect on the Buddhist story of the mustard seed. In the story, a married couple goes to the village holy person to ask for help. They have not been able to conceive and feel they have let down their families. They ask the holy person to help them in their deep sorrow. The holy person agrees to help but says that first they must collect a portion of mustard seeds. The couple is hopeful because mustard seeds are so common, but the holy person tells them the seeds must come from a family that has endured no pain from sickness, death, or financial problems. The couple enthusiastically sets off, visiting their neighbors in the village to collect the mustard seeds.

At the first house, a man offers to share some, but when the couple explains they cannot accept the seeds if anyone in his house has experienced sorrow, the man says, "Alas, I can't give you my seeds. Just this year my aunt developed cancer and has been very sick." So the couple thanks the man and moves on. The lady next door is happy to share some mustard seeds, but when the couple explains the rule, the woman says, "I'm so sorry, but in my house we are grieving the fact that my father just died." So the couple moves on. The family in the next house is happy to share their mustard seeds, but they are now bankrupt due to the collapse of their business. The couple moves on, visiting house after house in search of the seeds, but they cannot find a single person who has not experienced deep sorrow or pain. They return to the holy person, who asks them if they have returned for a solution to their pain. The couple answers that they no longer feel alone because they can see how much every family in the village has suffered.

It's easy in the midst of crisis to feel alone, as if yours is the 1 family on the block that is falling apart while everyone else is leading happy, impressive lives. The mustard seed story—and its message that all humans have had their share of suffering and crises—has been a comfort to me in difficult periods. What speaks to me, and might also speak to you, is another piece of hopeful news: Our circumstances and thinking can and will shift, as it did for the couple. With time, we will find ourselves feeling better. This gives me hope, and I hope it provides the same for you.

Final Thoughts

Although I usually include toolbox takeaways for each chapter, this is a topic for which I encourage you to look at the explanations and tips I provided for the urgent crisis you and your family may be facing. Do not ever hesitate to reach out to your doctor or mental health professional if you are worried, and keep the lines of communication open with your children as much as possible, no matter what. Ensure that you make your own self-care a priority during these rough times so you can be your child's best advocate. Remember, everyone has times when there are rough waters, but with help and support, most families will get through it strong. Keep your head up and remember—this too shall pass.

QUIZ

Does Your Child Have Tools to Find Their Purpose?

1. When it comes to your child's current after-school activities, they
   a. Typically seem eager to attend and are in a good mood afterward. They talk with enthusiasm about what happened at the practice/activity/lesson. (0 points)
   b. Periodically resist going and are sometimes relieved when it's over. (3 points)
   c. Must be forced to attend these activities. (5 points)

2. True or false: Your family has values that you have clearly articulated and repeated to one another.
   a. True! In fact, my kids can correctly name many of our family values. (0 points)
   b. Somewhat true. I think my child could name some values that we hold, especially if I gave them a little help. (3 points)
   c. False. We haven't really discussed our values. (5 points)

3. If you asked your child to name their strengths or talents, they

    a. Could easily and accurately name multiple strengths. (0 points)

    b. Could probably identify at least 1, although they may need help. (3 points)

    c. Would likely be at a loss. (5 points)

4. How often does your family pause all activities for purposeful downtime, conversation, or reflection?

    a. More than once a week (0 points)

    b. Once a week (1 point)

    c. At least once a month (3 points)

    d. A few times a year (4 points)

    e. Once a year or less (5 points)

Add up your score. Total _____

What Your Score Means

0 to 6 points: Your child has many of the tools that will position them to find joy and purpose in life. They have opportunities to pursue their interests, they have a set of values to fall back on when making decisions, and they find plenty of quiet time to reflect on their lives. The toolbox explored in this chapter will provide additional ideas to help them build on these successes.

7 to 15 points: We all want our kids to have a strong sense of self and drive to carry them through life, and your child has a good start. But like most kids, they could likely use some help exploring what motivates them and gives them joy. This chapter explores tools to help your child with these questions.

16 to 20 points: It's common for families to pursue the pre-scribed path set out by others in their community. It can be tempting to try to keep up with it all, but that is not easy and can be physically and mentally exhausting. In this chapter, we'll consider tools to help you and your child think about who they are and what motivates them. Thinking about those deeper questions can lead to happier, healthier kids.

CHAPTER 9

Giving Our Children Tools for Success and Happiness

Many of us as parents do our best to direct our kids on a path to success, but often it doesn't seem to stick. Are we doing something wrong? Why is it that our child is not excited about being on the football team or motivated to make good grades? Is it them, or is it our parenting?

What is it that leads a child to be happy and fulfilled in life?

Marla was 14 when she hit that proverbial wall. Her parents were ambitious and hoped that Marla, who had learned to read at the age of 2, would study medicine and perhaps even neurosciences as her dad had done. In ninth grade, Marla experienced a difficult time with math and chemistry and became more interested in writing and journalism. Her parents continued to push her in STEM (science, technology, engineering, and math) subjects until 1 day when she told them that that was not who she was. She joined the school newspaper and loved it. Her passion was journalism, and that was what she wanted to do.

Success envisioned by parents might be different from the success that your child might want. Success is largely in the eye of the beholder. Some children may naturally be inclined to be ambitious and competitive, and may seek a hobby or career within that passion, while others may be more motivated by creativity. For contentment in life, our children need to find and embrace their goals. If we force *our* vision of success on them, it may lead to a lack of happiness and self-confidence and even to resentment, which can affect our relationship with them. As parents, we are here to guide them—not force them.

Children have different personalities, and often our challenge is getting to know them well so that we can understand what motivates them and what may not. My daughter tends to be driven by challenging goals. She seeks out the toughest academic classes and strives to be pushed by us as her family and by others. That is where she finds her energy. My son is much more social and craves conversation and affection, even though he likes challenges, too. Understanding their different needs helps me to be a better parent.

For our kids to have a better chance to be happy and successful, there are certain elements that are important. I call them the *4 Ps*: purpose, principles, pause, and pivot.

The First P: Purpose

In the book *The Alchemist,* by Paulo Coelho, a boy goes on a journey to find his "personal legend" and finds happiness along the way. It's a simple story and has 1 main theme: Those who find a purpose or passion in their lives end up being fulfilled, happy, and often very successful, too.

In fact, from a scientific perspective, having a purpose or goal is associated with not just contentment psychologically but also better health physically. In several studies, having a purpose was associated with a lower risk of heart disease and stroke, longer life span, and better economic and financial status. The more often a person had short- and long-term goals, the happier, healthier, and more successful they were. It seems intuitive, but it's not easy to see this as parents. We often get stuck on the proverbial treadmill juggling our jobs and household duties, and carting the kids to and from 1 activity or another, without thinking about what the greater goal might be.

As parents, we are also often influenced by others in our community. When you hear about the girl in your child's class who has now joined a travel soccer team, you may be inclined to look into it yourself. No one wants to be left behind, but if your child feels the pressure more than enjoyment, it ends up being a loss of time and money and leads to frustration.

Three principles can help to decide whether an activity or a pathway is the smart choice for your child:

1. **Does this activity make your child feel fulfilled? Is it a step to an agreed-on goal or purpose?**

   If your tween or teen comes back from an activity excited and happy, chances are they like it. Of course, any activity or subject of study has its bumps and hard work, and this is something that should be discussed and, for the most part, accepted. Knowing and discussing a future goal together can help make the bumps easier. For younger kids, this may just be finding a hobby or activity they enjoy. For older children, the discussion can include whether the hobby or activity could be a potential career path either in college or as a profession. If there is no joy at all from something, it may be time to reconsider.

2. **Does this activity or subject play to a strength that you, others, or your child has identified?**

   Not everyone can be a great athlete, and not everyone can be a great musician, artist, or even scientist. Does this activity or subject build on talents that your child has? Have teachers commented on this as a strength in the past? Is it something that your child feels good about? Of course, if they enjoy it, then the activity could be a keeper.

3. **Does this activity, hobby, or subject of study help your child's self-worth?**

This again feeds into what feels right. One way to help determine this is to have your child ask the following question: Does it help me and/or someone else? One girl I know really enjoyed going to food banks to feed the hungry. She felt like she had done something good by helping others. This is, in turn, helped her nurture compassion, which eventually led her to start a club at her school to help the hungry.

Helping your child find their purpose and passion takes time. In fact, when kids are younger, around ages 4 to 8, it makes sense for them to try different activities so that they (and you!) can identify what seems to stick for them. It is a process, and it must be nourished and cared for, just as you would a garden. This means coming back to the table with your kids and having discussions about opportunities that may arise, as well as obstacles in the way. But having intentional and thoughtful ways to find a main theme or purpose is very important as a step toward your kids' happiness.

The Second P: Principles (and Values!)

Principles enhance your family members' lives and lead to contentment. This is another dimension of building the main theme of your child's life, and it feeds into purpose as well. Principles and values are intrinsic to your nuclear or extended family but also may be derived from community, such as a place of worship or even a team sport.

Principles or values can help shape a person's self-identity. The idea that certain areas define who a person is can help in situations they encounter and also help their self-esteem. "I am a kind person" or "I work hard to meet my goals" or "family is important to me" are concrete ideas that can help all of us, but especially our children, who are often in the limbo stage of deciding who exactly they are.

Education

Education might be 1 example of a family value. I was once asked by a friend why it is that certain cultures seem to succeed so well academically. I paused when she asked me that and started wondering whether this was true.

One value that may be prevalent in these families is a higher emphasis on education and academics. Some families start on the academic track quite young, placing their children into math programs at the young age of 4 or 5, and often teaching them multiple languages quite young as well. I grew up with a very similar value system; my report card was central to many family discussions, and if there was a B, the conversation would go on for many days, much to my chagrin. Academic achievement for me eventually became an ingrained value and something I strived for. This is not to say that a strong academic achievement should be a value in every family or for every child, but for me personally, having this value as part of my main story often helped me to refocus and reorder my priorities in high school and college.

Family, Religion, and Other Values

Other values of importance to people may be family or religion. These can be focal points, and being consciously aware of these can help remind people what is important to them, adding the benefit of prioritizing and also becoming a system that they can measure decisions against. Family and religion are 2 areas that can also contribute to connection and having a sense of community, both of which are so important for all of us psychologically. Having the support of a group of people, whether through a place of worship or a neighborhood gathering, and being able to give support to those people as well, helps stabilize us emotionally and also gives us a sense of belonging and purpose.

With my own children, I'm working to ingrain values, including a commitment to avoiding drugs and substance use disorder, no matter the societal pressures. We've had many discussions over the years about the hazards of drug use, as well as drinking too much alcohol, and not putting yourself in a position where you have lost conscious control of your own actions and thoughts. I'm hoping that this voice will be in their heads when they find themselves in situations where they need to make critical decisions, while also knowing that the family will always be there for them if they do stumble or fall short of expectations. Their father and I will always love and accept them, and they can always come to us without fear of rejection.

Open communication and honesty are other values our family has spoken about many times. I encourage my children to come to me with anything, and I promise to be calm, to listen, and to help find a solution with them. Instilling these principles early on will help in all areas of life, such as jobs, education, and relationships.

Imagine your child in college or even their first job when they have moved away for the first time. There will be times when they will need to reach for that inner value system to help guide them in decisions for relationships (work or personal) or even in times when they may simply have had a bad day. Having the ability to prioritize based on the governing principles they have adopted gives them a sense of identity and the ability to reach out for support when needed.

The Third P: Pause

In our constant on-the-go lifestyle, taking a pause is the most difficult thing to do but may be of the most value. By pressing the pause button, I refer to the ability to do the following:

- **Making and building time into schedules to rest.** Stopping and resting allows us to reassess the situation and whether we are on the right track, allows the mind to increase creativity and innovation, and allows us to gather our energy. Pausing is essential to our mental and emotional well-being.
- **Pausing to stop allows you to see if others may need help.** Giving to and helping others not only benefits them but also you as the giver. There is a biological release of feel-good hormones that happens when you lift someone else up. Building a pause into your child's schedule can help them learn the benefit of compassion; in time, they may be able to incorporate this into their schedule on their own.
- **Pausing to reassess our connections with others.** As parents, when we are on the go, sometimes the hectic pace can create havoc in the very relationships we need to support and fulfill us—those with our partners, spouses, parents, and friends. It is key for us to help our kids learn to pause and highlight this very important aspect of life.

I remember when my son was in sixth grade and had a school dance, a bar mitzvah, and a birthday party all on the same weekend. I decided to sit down with him to discuss how we would manage it all. Before we even discussed options, my son asked if he could opt out of all the events and just spend the weekend at home with me. It made me pause and reevaluate what was important—time to rest and recover. That weekend we hung out at home doing mostly nothing and enjoyed the extra family time. On Monday, my son was refreshed and reenergized to head into a new week. He had known what was best for him during a hectic time.

Pausing is certainly not easy and, just like anything else, needs to be learned so that it becomes a habit. Some ways I have done this myself are the following:

- Block times off the weekly calendar for myself and my kids. Just like anything else, this should be built into the schedule. This will help automatically find time to do nothing or simply hang out.
- Start meditating. This is a biological way for our brain to reset. We often have monkey brain where we jump from 1 thought to the other and are lured away from our focus, which can also affect our emotional well-being. It's important to focus on our breathing even for just 5 minutes.
- Build in some pause time regularly with friends or relatives who you don't get to see or talk to very often. Is it your stepdad who lives far away? Is it a friend from high school? This is for you as a parent but will remind you to do this for your kids as well, if it's in your life regularly.
- Encourage your kids, no matter what age, to take breaks: Point it out to them. For younger kids, if they've had a hectic week, this may be a built-in relaxation afternoon for them to just lie around the house. Encourage breaks from devices. For older kids and teens, this may be a built-in study break when you ask them to do nothing or go for a walk. Pausing helps all of us.

Pausing is described well in the story of a young student who was learning archery. One day, he asked his master, "Why must we pull back the on the bow to make an arrow go? Why can't we just push it?" The master replied, "The bow must be pulled back to gather energy and momentum. Only then will it go with speed and focus to get to its target."

Similarly, we must rest and pause to gather momentum. This helps us become energized and stronger so we can reach the goals we want faster.

The Fourth P: Pivot

As a parent, have you ever had a job where things didn't seem to go as you had wanted? Was it a place where you felt exhausted or demoralized? Or maybe it was a boss who didn't understand you no matter what you said or did? There are also relationships, as well as problems such as health issues, that can feel as if you are constantly hitting your head against the wall. These are times when persistence may be tried, but a pivot or a change in direction might be needed.

Such was the case with Tim, who had played baseball for 6 years and simply wasn't progressing. He eventually told his dad that he had started disliking it and the practices for almost 2 years. He would come back deflated from his practices and his games, regardless of whether the team won or not. His parents finally decided that perhaps a change was necessary. When they asked him if there was something else he wanted to do, his eyes lit up. Tennis. He had been watching Wimbledon and other matches and wanted to try it. Two years later, Tim was on the tennis team in high school and went on to play for his college team, too. Sometimes when 1 direction is not working, changing direction can make all the difference.

Teaching children the ability to pivot is a fine balance with teaching the lessons of perseverance and rigor. It is a thoughtful decision that must be made after looking at all the variables and having team discussions between you and your kids. Sometimes it is a decision that needs to be made and teaches kids that it's OK to change direction when trying to find your passion.

The Bonus Tool: Parental Patience

One other P that we could add to this list as a bonus for parents, and certainly deserves to be mentioned, is patience. This is so difficult sometimes, when we as parents are managing so much, but it is very important. I remember a parent sharing with me an argument she had with her daughter, Arielle. It was during the pandemic, and Arielle had been wearing a face shield to school every day, until she lost the shield. When her mom asked her where it was, Arielle said she didn't know. Arielle deflected her mom's anger by blaming the school, her brother, and even her mom for losing it. Her mom was astonished that Arielle wouldn't say she was sorry and accept responsibility, but after a huge argument, Arielle said, "If I say I'm sorry and say it's my fault, you will blame me for days. I'm scared to admit it was my fault." Listening and having patience can help us understand our children and their intentions better. Arielle's mom realized at that moment that she had to listen more to her daughter and to model patience. She made a pact with Arielle that she would have more patience and not place blame, as long as Arielle remained honest with her.

Toolbox Takeaways for Building Your Child's Success and Happiness

TAKEAWAY 1: **Strengths**

Using a sheet of paper, write down 2 to 3 strengths that you think your child has; then write 2 to 3 strengths that you perceive they see in themselves; and 2 to 3 strengths perceived in them by others, such as coaches, uncles and aunts, or friends. Ask your tween or teen to do the same. Compare notes and see what might be an area that they can build a passion or purpose in. This won't be one conversation; it likely will be many.

TAKEAWAY 2: **Passion**

When deciding about activities and whether they fall into the main daily schedule, ask your children how they want to spend their time. Remember pause time is a priority, as is family time, too. Is the activity something that your child is passionate about? Does it lead to the next step in their goals or purpose? Does it help others or align with your family's values or principles?

TAKEAWAY 3: **Habit**

If you decide to start meditation as a family, allow your kids to pick the music or app or even lead the meditation. Start with just 5 minutes, 5 days a week and grow from there. There are plenty of apps out there to help, and it may be difficult at first to make it a habit, but the rewards are astounding—better focus, better mood, and better health. And remember, it generally takes 21 days to form a habit.

TAKEAWAY 4: **Replenish**

When there is too much going on, and you feel as if you are driven by life, reassess. As a parent, you also need time to pause and replenish. If you are feeling stressed, chances are that your choices need to be reassessed and reprioritized. And that can mean saying no more often and choosing what deserves a yes.

TAKEAWAY 5: **Patience**

One of the most valuable tools, but sometimes the hardest when we are rushing, is patience. Patience and understanding require listening and considering other points of view. Even though it may be difficult at times, sitting down with your kids to understand their point of view and how their schedules are affecting them can go a long way toward fostering a strong relationship as well as finding peace and happiness for you and your family.

CHAPTER 10

Final Tools to Build Happy and Healthy Kids

Life is a journey with ups and downs, and the reality is that stress, positive or negative, will always be present in each of our lives. Our job as parents is to look for these stressors and assist in recognizing when our kids are overwhelmed, while teaching and guiding them to make the best choices that will benefit them emotionally, mentally, and physically. The reprioritization for our kids' mental, physical, and emotional health that I've discussed in this book, such as the stress relievers, the fundamentals, the importance of sleep, the resetting of schedules, and the critical key of replenishing yourself as a parent, can help reframe your and your kids' well-being and happiness.

Connection Through Community

Teaching our kids about the importance of connection through community is key in providing them with the buffers and the tools that they need to be happy. When you connect deeply with people, you build the safety net for when times are rough. Additionally, you have the opportunity to help others in your community by means of religious celebration, community service, or participation in neighborhood activities, while you are building a mental capacity to be giving and to care about others. That compassion and connection can activate parts of your brain that can chemically influence feeling good, too. When we hug, oxytocin is released, which gives us a happy feeling.

What matters is having a handful of deep relationships in your inner circle that give you the metaphorical life jackets to carry you when the seas are rough. I live very far from extended family, but every summer and during some holidays, we prioritize visiting with cousins. During the rest of the year, we prioritize socializing with several families in my inner circle, so my kids have "aunts" and "uncles" in our hometown, too, and feel that security.

The Power of Communication

We've heard it before—communication is one of the most important skills you can have in life. Whether you are in a relationship with friends or a partner, at work, or even with family members you have known forever, when you can't talk to one another, everything comes to a halt. Clear and respectful communication can make or break getting a job, a promotion, a desired grade, or even acceptance into the right school or college. So why not spend more time teaching our children to be good communicators? How can we add this to the toolbox?

This may sound cliché, but as parents, it starts with us. "Be the change you wish to see in the world" is a famous quote commonly attributed to Gandhi, a quote that we often refer to. Modeling good, calm, and honest communication is key for kids to learn how to communicate with their peers, with you, and with the world. I remember talking to a friend's son who shared that he had trouble communicating with his dad. Their family was going through some difficult times, and he thought his dad was hiding the truth. As a pediatrician and parent myself, I understood why his parents might not be being completely forthcoming with details about their jobs and livelihoods to their 11-year-old son. So how could they quell their son's fears, without hiding things from him? His parents and I talked about it, and they came to the conclusion that they could share details over time and that while their son didn't need to know everything, they assured him that they would always tell him the truth. Conversely, they would always expect the truth from him. For my own kids, I've told them repeatedly that honesty is what I expect, even if they think that the truth might make me upset. We have a verbal honesty contract. When appropriate, I often share with them things about my life to demonstrate what I expect from them. There will be times, when just like in any relationship, my kids may not want to talk. Or they have had a bad day and shut down. But this is true of adults, too. And just like we give our friends space when that happens, we can give our children that space as well, letting them know we are there for them when they are ready to share their thoughts.

Open and honest communication can also be a safeguard when your kids leave for camp, visit family, work a summer job, or attend college. The truth is, as parents, we cannot be with them every minute, making sure that they are safe. There will be times when they may be tempted to make poor decisions about issues such as substance use, digital devices, or even friends they decide to keep. Building and fostering a strong relationship based on trust and communication can be the safeguard your child needs. If something happens and they need a trusted adult to talk to, the chances are greater that they will come to you. And you will be there to help guide them through the choppy seas.

Self-esteem

Encouraging your children to communicate well with others is also an important tool to increase self-esteem. Share examples of how they can do so, whether it's talking to the basketball coach about how to improve their dribbling skills, their teacher at school about a missing assignment, or even responding to an email or text from a friend. Making communication skills a priority with siblings is also important. Every parent hopes that their kids remain close as adults. But laying down that foundation or pathway in their mind begins in childhood. There will always be disagreements, but it's just part and parcel of growing up. Teaching your kids to negotiate their points in a calm manner is very important and will not only help family relationships but also give them practice for making their point of view heard outside the family circle.

A friend's daughter, Alina, was upset 1 day about constantly being benched when playing hockey. No matter how hard she tried, she didn't have enough ice time when competing with another team. She thought she had improved and was very frustrated. Alina's mother suggested that she advocate for herself and speak to the coach. Alina and her mother practiced the conversation at home. At the next practice, Alina explained to her coach how she had worked hard and improved and deserved more ice time. To her surprise, the coach said he would give her more time and then they would reevaluate. By asking her daughter to communicate instead of stepping in and fixing the problem herself, Alina's mother had given her daughter a chance to advocate for herself and build the skills needed to promote self-esteem and confidence.

Communicating properly through various channels is an important part of this skill set, something that unfortunately schools don't necessarily have a curriculum on. For my own daughter in high school, learning how to communicate with her teachers respectfully, but confidently, on email has been a wonderful opportunity for her to practice in a safe setting. I have a rule at home that I have to see any emails my daughter wants to send, but only after she has worked on the first draft. Afterwards, she shows me what she has written in response. Then we edit it together before she sends it out. Giving them these opportunities coupled with your guidance can help them in the future with personal and professional relationships.

Gaining Clarity

The way we feel in a particular moment often influences the way we think and how we perceive situations. This can certainly influence how we react, and the same is true for our children. This is why it is so important to let our kids know that their mood or fatigue might be influencing how they react to a situation. Learning to recognize our current emotions and moods can help avoid knee-jerk reactions that may not be appropriate. Allowing our minds to cool down first allows us to see the bigger picture once those heightened emotions are no longer dominating the situation.

One way we can keep this lens clear is to build in a pause between an event and a reaction. An example of this from my own life comes to mind. I was having a very difficult time when my dad was hospitalized with a serious condition. He lived far away from me, and because I am a doctor, my family asked me advice about what should be done. I was extremely worried and stressed. Under these circumstances, when I received an email from a colleague, my mind immediately interpreted it negatively and I became upset. I was ready to shoot off a response, but thankfully I decided to pause and come back to it later. After hearing more positive news about my dad the next morning, when I went back to the email to respond, I was pleasantly surprised to find that the email wasn't negative at all. Taking the pause that the situation required allowed me to see it through a clear lens.

Compassion and Empathy

By understanding what others are going through and having empathy, we can connect to other people but remain grounded ourselves, comprehending the joys and the difficulties in life. Kids who volunteer to help may have the opportunity to see those who may not be as fortunate as they are. It helps to shift the question of "Why did this happen to me?" to "I am grateful for where I am and what I have." Empathetic concern, which is the genuine desire to help others, can activate the part of the brain that buffers the hormones released from stress. Clearing the lens can also be achieved with what many experts call viewing life with *equanimity.* This means the ability to stand back when life has its bumps and realize that this particular bump is 1 day of 1 year of many years and that it too will pass. Other ways to achieve this is through techniques such as mindfulness or visualization during challenging or stressful times.

Another tool that can help achieve clarity is one that often seems to be lost in our fast-paced lives, and that is simply finding quiet time. The act of having quiet or spaces of silence and time without distraction allows us to process events as well as reconnect with our intuition. Our intuition or gut has no scientific definition but often is the place where we are able to take all the information, digest it, and figure out solutions to our challenges. When we don't take this time for ourselves, we aren't able to activate that and can go through life being pulled by a runaway train rather than living with intention. Taking the time to pass along this skill to your own children will be rewarding in the long run.

I, too, have had to find ways to move through stress or grief, while still guiding my kids. When I experienced a very tough divorce during the 2020 pandemic, another difficult situation arose at the same time: My son and my father were hospitalized. During that time, I found myself often extremely sad, experiencing feelings of guilt and disappointment. In addition to my own struggles, my children also battled with their feelings from the tension in the home. We talked a lot together, and we gained a lot of knowledge and skills from a course called *Cognitively-Based Compassion Training* at Emory University, which helped us understand how to navigate these difficult times and emphasized how self-care was key. Though it's not always easy, now my kids and I use tools such as the pause between event and reaction, tapping into compassion for others, acknowledging gratitude, sharing our feelings, and even finding quiet moments to stabilize ourselves.

Prioritizing a Healthy Mindset

Mental and emotional well-being, and ways to sustain yourself in that zone of wellness, are very important for cultivating and achieving happiness and success. The tools in this book, along with the reset of what can help our children holistically, such as prioritizing nutrition, sleep, exercise, and scheduling in time to decompress, can make a real difference for you and for them in the future. Raising our kids to have healthy and happy lives is no easy task for parents. It takes thoughtfulness, planning, and understanding what is truly important. As stress levels continue to rise for most of us, it becomes even more important to reset, analyze what is important for our family, and make that happen. We can build happier and healthier kids, but it will take intention and goals, just like anything else. I hope this book has helped you with the tools to do just that.

Index

Page numbers followed by *f* indicate a figure.
Page numbers followed by *t* indicate a table.